CHALLENGES TO CONTEMPORARY MEDICINE

NUMBER SIX

BAMPTON LECTURES IN AMERICA

DELIVERED AT COLUMBIA UNIVERSITY 1953

CHALLENGES to CONTEMPORARY MEDICINE

by ALAN GREGG, *Vice President Emeritus
of the Rockefeller Foundation*

New York 1956 COLUMBIA UNIVERSITY PRESS

COPYRIGHT © 1956 COLUMBIA UNIVERSITY PRESS, NEW YORK

PUBLISHED IN GREAT BRITAIN, CANADA, INDIA
AND PAKISTAN BY OXFORD UNIVERSITY PRESS
LONDON, TORONTO, BOMBAY, AND KARACHI

Library of Congress Catalog Card Number: 56-12498

MANUFACTURED IN THE UNITED STATES OF AMERICA

Contents

1. How dear is life?   3
2. What is the meaning of disease?   25
3. Current factors affecting medicine   49
4. How are medical education and medical care best paid for?   77
5. The natural history of the doctor   100

CHALLENGES TO CONTEMPORARY MEDICINE

1. How dear *is* life?

THE Greek word for leisure was σχολή. From this source came the Latin word *escola* and eventually our word *school*. What a profound reminder of the Hellenic system of values that their word for leisure provided subsequent languages with the word for the place and exercise of learning!

Few—and I hope none—of the readers of these lectures will be under the pressure of "required reading" or the shadow of approaching examinations. It comforts me to assume that you are at leisure, not at school.

Since leisure provides the ideal cradle for curiosity and the perfect circumstance for reflection, I have chosen a subject that deserves your curiosity and your reflection. I have chosen to discuss the proper use of medicine and the medical profession, for I have become deeply concerned by the lag of the laity (and of some doctors) in understanding where the whole of medicine—Great Medicine, I would call it—belongs today. I am eager—but I hope not overeager—to offer interpretations, suggestions, reflections, surmises, and, in short, formulations that might help you. I added that I am not overeager because I am mindful of the sobering definition of a zealot as one who redoubles his efforts when he has lost sight of his aim.

The threads that will be found running through these

lectures are these: that medicine has made progress to a degree not now understood or appreciated; that it offers the means for modern man to have life and have it more abundantly; that it offers these means with such certainty and in such abundance that medical care (both preventive and curative) deserves to be held on a par with food, clothing, and housing as one of the essentials of keeping alive; that it is the prevailing concept of disease that determines how much and how wisely medical science and art will be used and added to; that serious and even threatening factors are now affecting the teaching and practice of medicine and medical research; that a way exists that would solve the cost of adequate medical care, medical education, and research; and that we must provide for the training and future careers of all the professions involved in curative and preventive medicine and in the rehabilitation of the handicapped if we wish to avoid a state of frustration bordering on disaster.

In slightly different terms, if only for the sake of clarity, the general argument is this: First, I want to call attention to how much more the whole field of medicine has done and can do for human life than is apparently realized. In fact, I shall examine some of the reasons for the apathy that discourages further advance. In the second chapter I shall present the theme that what man has done about disease derives to a remarkable degree from the interpretation he has set upon the existence of disease, or the way he explains it, and that changes are occurring today as we begin to embrace new interpretations of disease and health. The third chapter will contain comments on some of the powerful factors and influences that operate today upon practice, teaching, and research, such factors as prepayment plans, the growth of specialism, group practice, the paramedical professions, the increased length of medical education, the effects of the demands of military service, research and the growth of medical knowledge, and, finally, some of the effects of inflation. The fourth chapter will be devoted to the only way I see out of the difficulties now confronting Great Medicine, namely, voluntary health insurance on a much more rationally generous basis than our present ignorance and indifference now accord it. The fifth chapter will be devoted to what I would call "The Natural History of the Doctor." For although it is convenient to coin such abstract and collective terms as Great Medicine, we shall not understand the future of Great Medicine unless we understand the human beings who go into the medical and paramedical professions, and why and how they choose such careers.

Since this follows so closely upon the publication of the five volumes of the President's Commission on the Health Needs of the Nation and the "Report of the Medical Task Force of our Commission on the Organization of the Executive Branch of the Government," and since an enormous amount of diverse but interrelated facts and widely variant opinions are readily available to all, I have thought it impractical for me to make a digest, or a judgment, of so much current information. Consequently, I shall deal with a few subjects that have permanent importance rather than try to cover in detail many topics of medical interest. Events do not take place in a vacuum. Assumptions and current opinions have environments, too, and relationships often as significant as their recorded content.

When we use the phrase "run for dear life" or "work for dear life," we draw upon the forcefulness of a rather widely accepted view that life *is* dear. In such phrases we epitomize the assumption that survival is nature's first law. This law is so widely true that any exception to it—and there are such—calls for such stirring statements as "Greater love hath no man than this, that a man lay down his life for his friends." Thus the exception proves the rule—an aphorism, by the way, that was born when the verb "prove" meant "illustrate" —the point being that the exception illustrates the rule, which is a prettier thought by far than the imbecility of a false paradox.

Life is dear, and yet in the light of what medical science has accomplished in saving life and can continue to do, indeed, can increasingly do, it is perfectly reasonable to ask the somewhat sarcastic question, "Well, now, when it comes down to brass tacks and copper pennies, just how dear is life, after all? Is life so dear when we begrudge what strengthens it and lengthens it and sometimes saves it?" And do we know of anything that offers so much to life as does medical science wisely put to work for us?

Now, let us assume that there is in the world a definable and recognizable group of human beings who follow and apply a definable set of beliefs and practices to strengthen, lengthen, and save life. For the moment I will not give a name to these beliefs and practices. They have been both changing and growing over the past hundred years, and so has the training of the people who use them. Don't be impatient and force me to say that I am talking about the medical arts, and sciences and doctors and nurses and all of their teachers, leaders, and helpers. I want you to look afresh at the whole array.

In the war between the States, almost a hundred years ago, this group of persons, with their beliefs and practices, took care of the soldiers—both those who were wounded and those who were sick but not wounded. This they did

How dear is life? 7

also in the Spanish-American War, in the First World War, and in the Second World War. Let us contrast the success of their efforts by comparing the death rates, from disease, of men in service: where 650 men on the Union side died of disease in the Civil War, there were 250 in the Spanish-American War, 160 in the First World War, and 6 in the Second World War. An improvement of one hundredfold in 90 years.

Are there any possible explanations that would challenge the inference to be drawn from this remarkable gain in the control over disease? How could we doubt that these people who look after the sick have among their beliefs and practices something that works—and works for dear life? These are, however, not rhetorical questions. For if one could show that such improvement in mortality is not due to the advancement and improved application of medical knowledge but to nonmedical factors, then it is high time to find that out, prove it, and make it widely known that the claims of medical science are false. Let us, in short, be as certain as we can that the current statistics, whether military or civilian, apparently proving favorable changes in the incidence, duration, severity, and mortality of most of the known diseases can sensibly be credited to advances in medical knowledge and its application.

One could hardly take seriously any murmured suspicion that in every war the medical officers have had strong and continuing reasons for falsely reporting notable reductions in the number of deaths, or the number of seriously ill. An absentee from roll call is either sick, dead, or AWOL; and a man is either fit for duty or he isn't. The delivery of medical supplies and, in fact, the doctor's own personal status would suffer if his reports of sickness and deaths were notoriously suspect. There are too many checks and balances on the occurrence of significant falsifications of unverifiably optimistic records.

I have chosen the Army records to illustrate the improvement in our control over disease, but from civilian life the evidence might carry conviction even more cogently to my readers. In Chicago, for example, twenty-four years ago the cases of diphtheria reported were 6,012; four years ago there were 5. Twenty-four years ago there were 513 deaths among the 6,012 cases; four years ago there were no deaths among the 5 cases reported. Indeed, as the reporting systems for disease in civilian or military life improve over the years, and they undoubtedly have, illness is recorded more often as well as more accurately.

If several diseases seem to be occurring more and more frequently nowadays, we must remember that we are becoming better able to recognize them and less willing to allow illnesses to go unnamed or unproven. As more than one wise doctor has realized, the so-called rare diseases are a little commoner than they are reported to be, and the reports of the common diseases contain and hide rarer diseases. After Harvey Cushing had taught a generation of medical students in New England and elsewhere how to recognize and diagnose brain tumors, the reported incidence of brain tumors in New England and elsewhere increased. So, with the ever-increasing precision of diagnosis, we may expect diseases previously rare to seem to become more common, while the vast number of the undiagnosed sick and the obscurely ailing will be sorted and reported as having afflictions which have been present but which had previously been unrecognized or miscalled. When the headlines run "Doctors Here Discover New Disease," it does not mean that a new disease has been, as it were, concocted by nature to afflict the human race. It usually means either that a disease previously seen in some other part of the world has at last been recognized in these parts, or brought here. Or it may mean that after rather careful examinations and repeated experience some definable and oft-repeated pattern of signs and symptoms deserves now to be described, named, and in the future recognized for the separate disease entity it is. When a baby first begins to recognize various members of the family and differentiate between them, he is doing a similar thing. It is not quite so accurate to say that his acquaintances are themselves increasing in number as that his power of making acquaintances is increasing. The persons later to be known by him were in existence before he was born; but now he is learning to recognize them. So diseases are not increasing in absolute numbers, though it may seem so. Rather, it is that our acquaintance with them or our ability to recognize and record them steadily increases.

Then how does it happen that the death rate in the four wars I've mentioned has declined? Could it be explained by saying that in times gone by almost any young man, sick or well, was taken into the armed forces, whereas today we admit only the sturdiest, the healthiest, the least susceptible to infection, and those least likely to be harboring diseases communicable to others? Yes, that would partly explain the apparent improvement in the sickness rates. But then you will have to explain what enables us to select such paragons of health and exclude the rest. Obviously, the selection process that proves so remarkably advantageous is based not on luck but on physical examinations, which in turn are based on these same theories and practices I have been trying not to call medical science lest we lose the freshness of mind I want you to bring to the problem.

Maybe the apparent improvement is due to better nutrition, better housing, better clothing—in short, a higher standard of living and a better distribution of wealth throughout all classes of society from which soldiers were drawn for every war from 1861 to 1951. Maybe medicine is taking too much credit for itself.

Before the nutritional cause of pellagra was proven scientifically, pellagra was to be found even among the rich and persons with a high standard of living. Indeed, our ordinary housewife of today knows more about nutrition and useful dietary practices than did the most imposing medical authority in 1910. But she knows that, thanks to medical research. It has often been said that disease is no respecter of persons. I would edit that statement to read, "Disease is no respecter of persons who have no respect for disease—and the best source of respect for disease is an understanding of it." For it is still true that those diseases of which we have no substantial knowledge seem to be no respecters of persons. Undoubtedly, better nutrition, better housing, and better clothing make for better health and less disease all by themselves, but who supplied the standards by which one diet was found to be what is called "better" than another? Clearly, it was the physiologists, biochemists, public health men, and clinicians. Do we belittle medical scientists by borrowing their criteria to prove that medicine is not so important? I remember that A. G. Gardiner of the *Manchester Guardian* pointed out that the critics of Woodrow Wilson's mistakes in point of the League of Nations owed most of their standards of judgment to Woodrow Wilson.

Improvements in civilian housing can only in a few instances be advanced as bearing importantly on sickness rates of soldiers under field conditions. Indeed, getting used to no housing at all after being well housed is practiced deliberately and made more attractive by being called "hardening." And one may wonder how rapidly improvements in housing would have progressed if no medical scientist had been able to show that overcrowding produces ill health of various but specific and demonstrable kinds.

The argument that improvements over the years in the clothing of the population from which soldiers are recruited explains their better state of health possibly has some validity if one has in mind the large number of poorly-clothed persons fifty or ninety years ago. But since the recruits from the poor were given military clothing of uniform quality, at government expense, I would suspect that the improvement in the soldiers' health, if attributable to clothing, must be attributed to new types of clothing planned by hygienists and physiologists. What improved soldiers' clothing was a better knowledge of physiology applied to field conditions. Sunstroke among British troops in India was controlled more by the application of physiology than by increasing the clothing budget in British home populations or by expenditures for providing more red flannel underwear in the tropics.

In short, there is no sufficient reason for supposing that the reported improvement in the health of the human race or various parts of it over the past hundred years can be explained by claiming that the records are either falsified or misleading, or that improved general living conditions, which, incidentally, owe much to medical science and its applications, are in the last analysis mainly or immediately responsible. Before immunization was used, typhoid killed the well-dressed, well-fed, and well-housed. In the phrase "improvement in the health of the human race," I would include a reduction in the incidence of disease, a reduction of its severity, a shortening of its duration and convalescence, the alleviation of pain, a more frequent and more nearly complete restoration of function, a postponement of death—in short, a more abundant state of health and well-being from one end of life to the other and a lengthening of that span.

With this idea in mind of improving the health of the human race, let us look further. By the end of the first decade of this century, I think, enough precise, dependable knowledge was in the command of a large enough number of American doctors for there to be better than an even chance that one would be right in seeing a doctor for whatever disease one might have. Doubtless, well before 1910 some doctors were worth seeing regardless of what might be the trouble, not that they could help with all diseases or difficulties, but they had a chance of being useful—a chance that was worth taking. But by 1910 enough doctors had enough knowledge so that one could call a doctor at random and still probably do a little better than he would had he not bothered with a doctor at all. It is, therefore, a question not only of increases in medical knowledge but increases in the number of doctors well enough educated to know what to do and well enough trained to do it.

As an analogy, you can improve the batting average of a team of baseball players by raising considerably the batting average of a few players, or by raising a little the batting average of all the players, or by teaching some batters to knock home runs off some of the pitchers every time even if they can't hit other pitchers any better than before. Now, nature is quite a pitcher. She shoots a formidable variety of problems at the doctor.

The most compact and elegant statement of the progress of medicine that I know came from Lawrence J. Henderson when he said, "I think it was about the year 1910 or 1912 when it became possible to say of the United States that a random patient with a random disease consulting a doctor chosen at random stood better than a fifty-fifty chance of benefiting from the encounter." What Henderson was talking about was the batting average of doctors as a group. He didn't say that exactly in 1910 or 1912 every doctor could knock a home run, i.e., completely cure all or even 51% of his patients. He said that somewhere about that time the batting average of the generality of doctors had improved to a point where it made sense for one to ask them to go to bat. There are still plenty of diseases on which effective knowledge is nearly so completely, and therefore uniformly, lacking that one's choice of doctors should relate more to his capacity to learn than on his capacity to utilize what he already knows.

In point of the diseases we can't control yet, I often wonder why patients don't reckon five percent of their doctors' bills and send it to competent research agencies, since in the absence of improvement they could sensibly guess that they are in many instances not so much being treated for their disease as waiting for the right treatment to be discovered. For in a very real sense, many a patient is being simultaneously treated by two doctors, the one he goes to and the one who is doing some part of the research that will unsnarl the confusion or clear away the ignorance that is postponing the discovery of the right treatment.

Now, if Professor Henderson's reference to 1910 or 1912 as the time when the tide turned in favor of betting on the help of doctors, in other words, the beginning of the time when the odds were, broadly speaking, favorable for the patient, what can we say of the year 1956? The odds are almost immeasurably better. But let me begin the answer to that question by mentioning a few facts that may at the outset seem a bit remote.

One of the most curious and baffling results of the travel to some forty countries that I have done over the past thirty years in the study of medical education and research relates to what might be described as Lodge's law. Somewhere I saw a quotation from Sir Oliver Lodge to the effect that the last thing in the world that a deep-sea fish could discover would be salt water. In less picturesque language, the same idea can be phrased in the statement that it is always extremely difficult to be aware of what has always been and is still around you. In my experience, one can become aware of one's present environment best by leaving it for a while. And by the same token, an American traveler not only sees a new country with fresh and wide-open eyes, but on his return to America, or even before he has returned, he sees things in America he never noticed before.

So stimulating and refreshing has been this experience of discovering an America I would not have seen had I not left it that I would gladly pass on the discoveries. But I have found this bafflingly difficult. When in a Pakistani village that dozes in a tradition of two thousand years of somnolent sameness I find that the midwife gets three rupees if it's a boy and two if it's a girl, I suddenly sense a surge of novelty. For the first time I become aware that we assume in America a large measure of equality between the sexes.

How dear is life? 15

I realize that though such a degree of equality is by no means confined to America, it is so continuously taken for granted here that we cannot realize its existence. No traveler can ever convey the completely routine and binding character of some custom governing a foreign culture by merely relating it to friends on his return. The custom which is being related has to his incredulous audiences the status of being an exception: as an anecdote it fails to convey any flavor of the universality or the completeness of its acceptance in the other culture—which, after all, was its most impressive aspect. This suggests an interesting generality, namely, that in order to learn something vividly you should be in the minority and, thus, overpowered as well as informed. Such a hypothesis would explain the handicap of many a lecturer: his audience is not in the minority and hence is rarely overpowered. Quite evidently, he is in the minority and often overpowered. My hypothesis would also explain the frequent observation of teachers that they learn from their classes. And it is almost certainly the reason why those who understand best the problems of minorities in this country are those who at one time or another have lived themselves for a while as a member of a minority in some foreign country.

In leading up thus to some comments on the "salt water" that surrounds us here in America in point of the unconscious assumptions that have always surrounded us, I have the task of alerting you to your own unconsciously accepted ideas regarding what medicine can now provide in terms of prevention, alleviation, and cure of disease. In so doing, I run certain risks I don't relish. You may think me waxing lyrical about commonplaces, trying to dramatize the veriest routine, crying out "Jerusalem!" at the first dusty hamlet on the road, or otherwise draping very ordinary lay figures with silken theatricalities. But the fact is that using the eyes of a newcomer I want to draw your attention to what I see in the present state of medical science and medical practice.

What I see of greatest importance is that the immense progress of medicine in the past hundred years has come from the advancement of precise and dependable knowledge. Progress in the next hundred years will continue to depend on gains of precise and dependable knowledge. Such knowledge is necessary but not sufficient. We must also face the fact that we seem to understand neither the accomplishments nor the potentialities of medicine and are unwilling, therefore, to pay for it.

Our "salt water" is the value of good medical care. As I have remarked before, the casual apathy of the prosperous disturbs me.[1] We all have each his own formulation of what is the essential difficulty in the world today. My formulation, in broadest terms, would start with the assertion that we all face a peculiarly unfamiliar problem, namely, how to survive prosperity. Science and technological applications of science produce some things we all want—power, wealth, and leisure. Having had for millenia the task of surviving adversity, we place an unreflecting amount of confidence in power, wealth, and leisure, because they seem to answer so many of the afflictions of adversity. But now comes the scientist's contributions, and machine manufacture, mass production, and an extraordinary quickening and facilitation of communication, travel, and transport. All these

[1] William V. Houston, W. Albert, Jr. Noyes, Curt Stern, Alan Gregg, and Wendell H. Camp, *The Scientists Look at Our World* (Philadelphia, University of Pennsylvania Press, 1952), p. 93.

produce the wealth, power, and leisure that make up what we call prosperity. And leisure, wealth, and power, on either side of the Iron Curtain, raise the problem not so much of how to get them as what to do with them after we have them. To paraphrase a Chinese proverb, "To share poverty is easy; to share wealth, difficult."

The human race has had long experience and a fine tradition in surviving adversity. Many of the virtues we praise, and the distilled wisdom we venerate, relate to the survival of adversity. But we now face, as Thomas Nixon Carver pointed out, a task for which we have but little experience or tradition, namely, the task of surviving prosperity. However, we are not at sea; we come nearer to describing the actual situation by saying that our boat is shooting a cataract. The sequence has been: Curiosity has found knowledge, knowledge has led to power, power has provided wealth and leisure. Now leisure invites still wider curiosities. Prosperity may be the end of adversity, but it is not the end of living.

Among the problems of surviving prosperity, few are more baffling than the problem of keeping awake, staying alert, and remaining energetically responsive and responsible. Exactly on this point I should again raise the question "How dear is life?" for it seems to me that we do not realize how much medical research has won for us, how precariously we depend on medical education to preserve and perpetuate those gains, and how extensive, indeed, revolutionary, are the gains ahead if we recognize the newest problem confronting the human race, "How does one survive prosperity?"

For what may seem a prosperous and triumphant advance will entail new and unexpected problems. As an example, the advances of preventive medicine bring population problems to the fore. Not merely the quantity but the quality of the population comes into question—I hardly know which aspect of the population problem is the more important. Neglect of the quantity will bring the likelihood of war; attention to human genetics would seem to me likely to bring more improvement to human life than anything I know.

There is still and will probably long continue to be a sentiment akin to fear on the subject of research. No one has phrased this better than Freya Stark.

> In the West, spasmodically and with uncertain hands we try to eliminate the causes of sorrow; but it is only recently and since the decline of formal religion. The East still holds religion in its established forms: and encourages philanthropy which deals with effects and not with causes. For as soon as you investigate and try to alter the origins of things you are no longer a philanthropist but a revolutionary, and your disinterested movements are liable to make whole edifices crumble; and mankind is asked from successive pulpits to leave the fundamental things alone.[2]

Until we are convinced how great has been the advance thus far in medicine, I cannot expect us to sense the importance of retaining and maintaining it. Rather than exhaust the reader with statistics, I shall offer a few instances that contrast the past with the present.

Charles II of England died in 1685 after four days of serious illness. Loren MacKinney gives the following account of what was done for His Majesty, and I would call your attention not only to the bewildering variety of the measures employed but also to the fact that no record ap-

---

[2] Freya Madeline Stark, *The Southern Gates of Arabia* (London, John Murray, 1940), p. 143. Quotation used by permission of the publisher.

pears of any tests to determine the nature of the King's illness.

Once upon a time a king, while shaving, fell unconscious in his bedroom. The following treatment was employed by the royal physicians. A pint of blood was extracted from his right arm; then eight ounces from the left shoulder; next an emetic, two physics, and an enema consisting of 15 substances. Then his head was shaved and a blister raised on the scalp. To purge the brain a sneezing powder was given; then cowslip powder to strengthen it. Meanwhile more emetics, soothing drinks, and more bleeding; also a plaster of pitch and pigeon dung applied to the royal feet. Not to leave anything undone, the following substances were taken internally: melon seeds, manna, slippery elm, black cherry water, extract of lily of the valley, peony, lavender, pearls dissolved in vinegar, gentian root, nutmeg, and finally 40 drops of extract of human skull. As a last resort bezoar stone was employed. But the royal patient died.[3]

Bezoar stones enjoyed for centuries a legendary reputation as a sure antidote against poison. They were concretions or hard lumps of material formed in the alimentary organs of certain ruminants, especially goats.

A hundred years after the death of Charles II the reliance placed on bleeding and purging, under the authoritative advocacy of Benjamin Rush, had considerably increased.

Great as have been the changes in diagnosis and treatment over the past few centuries and, indeed, over the past few decades, we can well remain on guard against drawing universally optimistic conclusions as to the value of each new method while it struggles for recognition and authority. Rather than feel superior to the Philadelphian authority Dr. Samuel Gross (1808–84), in his statement that if the

[3] Loren C. MacKinney, *Early Medieval Medicine with Special Reference to France and Chartres* (Baltimore, The Johns Hopkins Press, 1937), pp. 33 f. Quotation used by permission of the publisher.

patient were bled less than sixteen ounces he was likely to feel cheated, we could more wisely reflect upon something far deeper, the power of authority, prestige, and custom in influencing methods of treatment. Excessive purges and blood letting as forms of treatment are fortunately things of the past but the psychological reasons for their one-time vogue may be continuing in some other guise. Let us remember that circumstances of obvious mortal danger have always tended to invoke tradition and authority with which to combat uncertainty, blame, or failure. It is to life's crises that we find, in almost any culture, the oldest customs and usages cling, and it is with these same traditional and often irrational procedures that preventive medicine has had to push statistical facts against the age-old belief that we *must* do something and preferably what has been done in the past.

From the ignorant zeal applied to the treatment of the sick or injured individual, let us turn to the ignorant bewilderment with which communities faced epidemic disease. Take cholera as an example—a disease now completely understood, or at least well enough to be under control.

From about 1816 cholera had been moving west from India. It was recorded in Moscow and in the Near East by 1830. Swiftly indeed, cholera was spreading to Western Europe, England, and Ireland. By 1832 an emigrant ship landed at Quebec with a record of deaths at sea from cholera among the passengers. Perhaps I can bring that event nearer by mentioning that two of my childrens' ancestors were buried at sea from that very ship four generations ago. Cholera spread to Montreal and thence to Albany, New York, Philadelphia, Erie, Buffalo, Detroit, and westward. By July 20 there were over 30 dead among the soldiers at Fort Dearborn. Those who could escape the afflicted cities fled, often taking with them persons already infected. By November, 1832, the deaths in Cincinnati had reached three hundred in about three weeks. The next spring cholera increased in its range and its ravages almost throughout the Mississippi Valley.

In these days of relative safety and protection we can recapture but little of the panic and terror that accompanied epidemic disease not much more than a century ago. In place of a joint resolution in Congress for a day of prayer introduced by Henry Clay, we have the more costly credits voted for the work of the United States Public Health Service. How fortunate is our generation!

I trust these records from the past make clear the substantive gains of modern medicine. But in a very different direction, namely, the future, I can see some less tangible but nonetheless valuable gains—gains that liberate the human spirit. Medicine is a broad field, indeed, and in it is to be found a special sector called, I think a little narrowly, psychiatry. It deals, among other things, with the study of man's mind and emotions. It is a field of medicine with many handicaps: it has profited less than several other medical fields from the scientific methodology of the last hundred years; animal experimentation offers less direct help to the solution of its problems than to the problems of infectious disease; mental disease affects human relationships intimately and powerfully, and thus both theory and practice in psychiatry offer obstacles of extreme complexity. Nonetheless, if I may be excused, I would state again my reasons for considering the future of psychiatry important:

> First, psychiatry along with the other natural sciences leads to a life of reason. It explains what must otherwise excite fear, disgust, superstition, anxiety, or frustration. It breaks the clinches

22 *How dear is life?*

we otherwise get into with life and all the unnecessary, blind infighting.

In the second place, by showing us the common rules, the uniform limitations and liberties all human beings live under because they are human, psychiatry gives us a sort of oneness-with-others, a kind of exquisite communion with all humanity, past, present, and future. It is a kind of scientific humanism that frees us from dogma and the tyranny of the mind, a relief from the inhuman strait jacket of rigid finality of thought.

Third, psychiatry makes possible a kind of sincere humility and naturalness I've never received from any other study or experience. . . . It provides the material for a sympathy that is honest and eager. . . .

I didn't mention the rewards research offers to human curiosity. Nor the satisfaction of being of help to poor, battered, dependent, frightened people and the justice of giving them the breaks just for once. Nor the immense economy of patching lives to a point of meeting life's demands. Nor the hope that we may understand what disease connotes as well as what it denotes. Nor the possibility that through psychiatric understanding our successors may be able to govern human politics and relationships more sagely.[4]

Obviously, more extensive and perhaps, therefore, more compelling as a subject for speculation is the comprehensive view of all the fields of medicine which are likely to be thrown open for cultivation and a rich harvest in future years. I often think how sorry our descendants a hundred years from now will be for us in our struggles put forth today in error and in ignorance, "toughing it out," knowing so little that is true and so much that isn't true, in the light of knowledge that will be commonplace in 2056 A.D.—if we will have passed on the torch to our children.

If we now have control over most of the infectious and parasitic diseases, if our knowledge of nutrition and general

[4] William C. Menninger, *Psychiatry in a Troubled World* (New York, The Macmillan Company, 1948), p. xiv.

hygiene already makes the sense of well-being not uncommon even for people over sixty years of age, if this knowledge has made possible a life expectancy of over 67 years for both males and females, if we have found in research the discovery of the method for future discovery, if we are on the edge of finding such laws of heredity as will enable us to profit from the innumerable experiments of nature effected by the "dance of the chromosomes," and if the understanding of the emotional and intellectual life of man is to be added to our present control of his environment, does not provision for the use and growth of medical care deserve an equal place with food, housing, and clothing as one of the essentials of keeping alive?

How dear do we really hold life if we begrudge the medical schools the cost of preparing the doctors to protect ourselves, our children, and their children? How dear do we hold life if we aren't prepared to set aside as much as a hundred dollars per capita a year as insurance against illness? How childish to pity ourselves for having to suffer so-called catastrophic illness when what turns illness into catastrophe is our catastrophic improvidence! And yet our medical schools are languishing for the lack of financial support, and our hospitals are all but apologetic for the dearness of dear life, and we shudder as we read exhaustive reports on the cost of medical care, as though the ideal would be to have no care at all when we need it. The ideal would be to have no need for medical care, and yet we do not take anywhere near all the steps we could to prevent disease.

If Americans each set aside $100 a year for sickness insurance, we should have sixteen billion dollars for education, research, medical care, and the very preventive measures that would reduce the need for medical care. Now, I own and operate two hats a year, one felt and the other straw. They cost about $15 each, and before the year is out I presume I spend another $15 each in checking them in hotels and restaurants and having them blocked and cleaned. Thus the cost of a conventional but unnecessary article of clothing comes to about $60 a year. If this seems liberal to the point of extravagance, I'll be more frugal in naming another expenditure. The laundry of but three shirts a week at 25 cents each, plus the purchase of one shirt a year at $6. My bill for one shirt, two hats, and the washing of three shirts weekly for a year amounts to $105. Why all this naïve petulance about the cost of medical care?

Medical science, with an additional sixteen billion dollars to draw upon, could give a service the like of which has not ever been known, a service of a thoroughness, convenience, and efficacy such as to reduce the incidence, the severity, and the cost of present illness in our population. How dear is life?

2. What is the meaning of disease?

IMPERCEPTIBLE as the earliest stages of some diseases may be, the sensation of being sick is usually convincing, and the majority of illnesses are accompanied sooner or later by symptoms or signs that are obvious enough. Subjectively feeling sick, even if it is no more than nausea, warns us that our state of being has changed. Pallor or weakness or slowness of response and movement, examples of signs readily observable by others, lead to the same general conclusion, namely, that our normal state of well-being can change or be changed into another state so obviously different as to demand attention. Probably, therefore, from the earliest days of articulate human thought there has been some word for, or concept of, disease as a state of affairs in certain contrast to that of health or well-being. Obviously, pain has always been more clamant and arresting than the general feeling of sickness, but it would seem likely that, since pain is always to some extent localized, the very experience of pain may have retarded somewhat the development of the concept of disease as a change affecting the whole being. As anyone knows, general malaise, or, in the less elegant vernacular, "feeling rotten," is a more pervasive and disturbing experience than many kinds of pain.

Resorting reflectively to distant lands or to distant periods in human history, we eventually encounter not only different diseases but something which is perhaps less obvious but more surprising than the mere diseases themselves. We encounter widely variant attitudes taken toward disease. By attitudes I mean the interpretations put on the mere existence of disease, the meaning of disease as a general phenomenon, how it is to be taken, how explained, and the position which the fact of disease occupies in the general scheme of things.

Quite characteristic of the habit of the human mind, we seem to find considerable comfort in interpreting an experience if we can find a plausible or even generally accepted cause for it. If we think we know its cause, in some measure we are at least relieved. Likewise, we take similar solace from giving it a name even when thinking about the name might raise more questions than it answers. At all events, both history and travel, or the lessons to be learned from excursions into both time and space, make it quite evident that the way man has chosen to think about disease has been, and continues to be, of quite extraordinary, and yet often ignored, importance. Indeed, there is such an intimate relationship between what we *think* about the fact of disease and what we are inclined to *do* about disease that I am disposed to think that what we do about disease shows the core and kernel of what we think about it. Of course, thought and action are not the same: one has only to add honesty to laziness to admit that thought and action are neither identical nor equivalent. But thought is so often inarticulate and inexplicit, whereas action is so much easier to observe, record, and remember. So, with certain safeguards and reservations, one is justified in inferring how men have thought about disease by noting what they have

What is the meaning of disease? 27

done about it. And certainly if we could obtain and spread a new way of thinking about illness and suffering, our conduct would tend in the aggregate to change as a result of such a new-found idea. To answer the question, "Where does medicine belong today?" one must examine the various successive but overlapping and interdigitating interpretations of the meaning of disease as they have occurred in the past or as they still exist in different countries today.

Now, in the initial experience of every human infant, cuddling and punishment, companionship and loneliness, protection and desertion, tenderness and violence, usually come from other human beings. It is only natural, therefore, to suppose that primitive man had a tendency, derived from such experiences, to attribute the discomforts of disease to the action or the intent of others. Primitive man's assumption that there are in addition to persons you see spirits you don't see was doubtless made easier by the fact that he didn't have eyes all around his head, and by the nontransparent character of rocks, trees, hills, and clouds, which hid things from his sight. The ordinary housefly, with an amazingly inclusive field of vision, probably has a harder time accepting the idea that the unseen exists; for him, probably, danger lies in what approaches, not in what is outside his field of vision. But for man danger *lurked*, and spirits nevertheless existed, even though they were not seen, and injury came from the will of others. In any event, the belief that disease comes from evil spirits or hostile persons has been found widespread; and apparently it has been so from time immemorial. The course of communicable diseases frequently gave support to such a view of the cause of disease. We still speak of "catching" a cold from someone or "giving" it to someone else, and epidemics, as we observe, spread and, as we say, "attack" us. In days gone by the terrifying suspicion of the personal malevolence of witches was turned into conviction by the testimony of the accused under threat of torture or in torture itself. Thus fear furnished the alphabet, as it were, to spell out the meaning of disease. Nor was fear the only misleading guide. Guilt and its demand for sacrifice or expiation has for thousands of years misled our poor human minds in deciding what to do about illness. Indeed, I have often marveled that the human race ever issued from the quicksand of fear, the quagmire of guilt, and the Slough of Despond that superstition set in the way of the sick and suffering. Nor have fear and guilt quite left the scene today: witness the common attitude toward mental disease. One can hardly regard superstition about disease as entirely a thing of the past. It were better to seek its relics and reminders in our present attitudes, for there are such remnants of superstition still awaiting intelligent attention. In many an anxious patient the shadow of possible guilt flits in and out of his resentful question, "But why should this happen to *me?*"

When disease was believed to come from the malice, the hostility, or the disfavor of other persons or of evil spirits, what was done about it? Flight is, of course, one of the primal reactions to attack. Moving from one locality to another has long been one of the commonest reactions to illness or even the fear of it. My own parents left Hartford, Connecticut, in 1882 for Colorado because of the frequency of malaria in Hartford. But to return to a larger segment of human behavior, when flight was impossible or inexpedient, the feasible alternative was to seek for the help at hand in the usual alternative to flight, which is fight. Healthy persons were called in as allies against further malevolence. This assistance came, in the earlier stages of illness, very naturally and most commonly from parents, relatives, dependents, and friends, and in varying measure and mixture, proffered or invoked.

Besides this rather heartening example of sympathy and mutual aid, a further action was taken, an additional maneuver which bears even today on therapeutic relationship: there was an almost universal tendency to formalize the status of some member of a group or clan into that of a professional medicine man, shaman, or healer. In the obvious emergency of illness it would be intolerable to have no one to call on, no one deserving a measure of confidence in some fashion appropriate to the occasion, no one ready to supply stability and authority in a situation whose terror and anxiety would increase in the presence of indecision and unstructured mediocrity.

Thus, in the earliest procedures devised to deal with disease, we see that somebody is chosen to take the acknowledged burden of the healer. The doctor is all but created by the patient and his anxious relatives and friends. Nor is this all. They want their healer to be remarkable. If the healer looks unusual, acts not as other men, and speaks incomprehensibly, wonder may willingly turn to awe and respect. His patients are more than willing to believe him perfectly exceptional: they want to believe their savior quite irreproachable. His remedies, too, may well be bizarre, exotic, astonishing, and rare. He can well hold himself somewhat aloof. For it is no fun to be in a desperate crisis with no one of exceptional talent, skill, and power to match the extremity of your need. Haniel Long has written a remarkable study of this relationship in a little book called *The Power Within Us*.[1] In superstitious terror a frightened patient and his anxious friends resort quite understandably to passionate and irrational credulity. We can hardly wonder, then, that medicine men through the ages have availed themselves of the peculiar status thus pressed upon them. Nor can one be much astonished if the medicine men took themselves at times at a valuation insisted upon by those in trouble. Indeed, because of the inherent tendency of the organism to survive many diseases—long called the *vis mediatrix naturae*—the subsequent recovery of the patient could surprise even the medicine man himself and at times convince him that he possessed more than natural powers or ordinary wisdom. Also, from this earliest view of disease came, as it seems to me, today's implicit assumption that essentially the doctor must be the ally of the patient, or at times his dominating guide, but not a servant, nor a judge, nor an antagonist, nor a moralizing critic, nor a policeman, nor even, indeed, an ordinary fellow mortal, as fallible as many and as imperfect as all.

Another important accompaniment of the assumption that disease is a misfortune willed or imposed by persons or spirits was the uneasy suspicion that it might at times be a well-deserved punishment. For this reason superstitious guilt feelings often complicated the earlier concepts of disease. And, of course, if the list of taboos were long enough, and if the highly detailed rituals and observances involved enough complications of timing and method to provide a manifest margin of probable infringements, errors, omissions, and failures to keep exactly to the prescribed rules,

[1] Haniel Long, *The Power Within Us*. (New York, Duell, Sloan, & Pearce, 1944).

What is the meaning of disease? 31

then the medicine man had all that he needed to say, "I told you so! You didn't follow exactly what I told you. You had it coming to you!"

Between this concept of disease held by primitive man and that portrayed in the Old Testament, the principal difference seems to me to be that the ancient Jews looked on disease as the evidence of the disfavor of but one God, and an all-powerful one, rather than the individual and isolated malice of minor deities or unidentified spirits. Such disfavor of God Almighty could come for reasons inscrutable, or for reasons already all too heavily weighing on the conscience of the afflicted. Whereas a North American shaman could exorcise, or expiate, or intercede with, a single evil spirit in behalf of a client without enraging any other gods, it must have been hard for the priests under a monotheistic system to run any risk whatsoever of seeming to criticize, or stay, or even mollify, the punishment obviously meted out to a sick man by the very same Jehovah everybody feared. From such an absolute interpretation of disease there was no escape but tears at that epitome of impasses, the Wailing Wall. The depth of the confusion and bewilderment occasioned by illness held to be due to divine disfavor has, I hope, no equal in medicine today.

In really striking contrast to such animistic or theological interpretations of disease came the contribution of the Greeks. I often wonder if the deep significance of the rationality of the Greek mind was appreciated or even realized in its time. As applied to medicine, much of the change to a more rational view of illness came from the Greek interpretation of disease as a lack of wholeness or harmony. To capture the refreshing sanity, impersonality, detachment, equanimity, and practicality of the Greek interpretation of disease, let me invent a completely modern analogy. Consider the state of one's emotions and thinking when a front tire blows out, (1) if it is believed that some unseen enemy has willed or contrived to have it blow out, or (2) if it is believed that it is God's way of showing His displeasure that your last contribution to the church showed a picayune appreciation of His blessings during the last twelve months, or (3) if it is explained that the front wheels have been for some time in need of realignment, and for that reason the tread wore thin. It is clearly the last interpretation that promises the largest measure of progress in increasing one's knowledge of the care and maintenance of automobiles, for it puts one in command of the situation. That is the important point: the purpose of all good therapy is to put the patient in command of the situation.

So great was this Greek contribution to medicine that it is by no whim of chance that our medical terminology is so largely Greek in origin, that we call the essential method of medical reasoning the Hippocratic method, and that as heirs to so remarkable a heritage we choose to bind ourselves with the Hippocratic oath. For, following the Greeks, we now take disease to be an entirely reasonable process, obeying laws eventually patent to observation and to reasoning. There are exceptions, perhaps, to so categorical a eulogy of the Greek interpretation of the nature of disease. I doubt, for example, whether the Greeks maintained quite so detached, rational, and naturalistic a concept of mental diseases or epilepsy. But even if the Greeks had managed to be to some extent rational about insanity, the demoniac possession theories prevailed in later centuries. But in the main, the immense advantage of the Greek view was that, in the relative absence of superstition and fear, it built, with its amazingly rational approach, at least the scaffolding for the advancement of knowledge.

Then came a new set of ideas about disease. The growth and spread of the Christian faith added a fresh component to the interpretation of illness and suffering. This is epitomized in the name of one of the famous hospitals in Paris, L'Hôtel Dieu—God's Hostel. The argument, so to speak, ran something like this: If Paradise awaited the suffering, then was it not evident that they were the elect of God, and was not association with them an act of recommended mercy inviting divine approval? "Misericordia" remains upon the name plates of thousands of hospitals in the Latin countries of two continents; and Lazarus became a saint. Gone entirely was the suspicion that you were interfering with divine punishment in consorting with the sick. To the contrary, it was courting divine favor and forgiveness to help the sick, indeed, merely to associate with them, even with lepers and the insane. Witness the Misericordia in Florence or the town of Gheel in Belgium, two monuments of the Christian interpretation of illness that are remarkable to this day.

With such an interpretation set upon disease, collections of the sick known as hostels and hospitals came into being, and an unprecedented opportunity thus came to hand for comparing the symptoms and signs of one patient with those of another. It does not matter that such an opportunity came into being without any foretaste of what it would do for medicine. It derived simply and directly from a new concept of the meaning of disease. And then a quite unexpected factor came into play.

In the halls full of sick persons, comparisons were inevitable. So easy were comparisons that differentiation, broad groupings of similarities, and, with the slow passage of time, the recognition and description of separate disease entities occurred, thanks in large measure just to the collection of patients in hospitals in the name of God. The debt of medicine to this by-product of a change in interpreting disease is not confined to the Christian religion. But Christian charity has helped the growth of medicine for upwards of a thousand years, and its advantages to medicine are easier to imagine than to define. There again, it is not the change in the incidence or the character of disease that deserves our attention, but rather the change in the meaning attached to the fact of disease. That is the point to notice.

I would not be misunderstood as implying that Christian hospitals produced immediate or rapidly improving gains in medical knowledge. The minds of physicians were bound for centuries by the authority of Galen and the conservatism of the church. Indeed, until the gains of medical science, at first halting and disputed, but in the nineteenth century vigorous, prolific, and self-evident in their efficacy, became available, the hospital was a rather terrifying blend of poorhouse and pesthouse, a place to die in, and a last resort in nearly every sense. In some ways one could suspect that the hospital served better the fears and consciences of those who were well than it met the needs of those who were sick. We do not have to look too diligently to find similar motives controlling the actions of those who located asylums for the insane well away from centers of population—and that not too long ago.

For centuries medicine was practiced with dumb empiricism and stubborn hope interwoven with over-systematized speculation, Galenic authority, and religious dogma. Then very slowly there began a new development in the way disease was regarded.

What is the meaning of disease? 35

What we are pleased to call the refinements and advances of making war began, even if slowly, to change our attitudes, first toward injury, and eventually toward disease. Because wounds were so obviously mechanical, man-made, and of every grade of severity, the lightest causing only a temporary loss of fighting ability, military surgeons were encouraged to deal mechanically to restore tissues and structures injured mechanically. Perhaps even more important, the military doctor's services began to be regarded in at least the faint glimmering light of having actual military value. I say the faint glimmering light, since, until the nature of sepsis and infectious disease were scientifically understood, the military doctor's services were small, indeed, in the maintenance of military strength. But by almost imperceptible changes at first, and later by conspicuous advances, disease and injury have come to be regarded as avoidable losses of military strength, and health has consequently come to be held as a means to an overwhelmingly important end. As an outgrowth of this view of disease, the records of physical examinations of young men drafted for military service have attracted attention and at times aroused concern over the state of health of the nation viewed in terms of strength. We could summarize this transition by observing that disease is no longer a mark of divine election but a threat to the national welfare.

I wonder whether anyone has just now noticed a remarkable word in the preceding sentence? The word is "national." Now, that word refers to a political concept no older than the French Revolution yet so constantly about us today as to suggest the salt water of Lodge's deep-sea fish. Let me suggest the relative novelty of the concept of nation by saying that last year in India I was told that when the constitution of India, which was drafted first in English, came to be translated into Hindustani, there was no word in Hindustani for "nation." It interests me that as old an art as healing finds support and even justification in being associated with as new a concept as that of nation—national welfare.

Indeed, this change can hardly be regarded as the contribution of the military alone, for Disraeli, with a considerable degree of imagination or prescience observed, about a hundred years ago, that the greatest wealth of a nation was the health of its citizens.

But military men have had, and have used wonderfully, an opportunity to demonstrate the value of certain medical measures on a scale and with a measure of control not easily applied in civilian life. The proof of the efficacy of measures for the prevention of yellow fever by mosquito control in Panama was possible in a way that could hardly have been accomplished anywhere at that time without military discipline and thoroughgoing mass-measures. F. F. Russell's demonstration of the value of inoculation in the prevention of typhoid both derived from and contributed to the belief that disease is an avoidable loss of strength in an army, and in a nation as well as in an individual. Such a view of disease receives the more weight from the number and power of the resources it calls into action; instead of being offered to the advantage of a privileged few, it is made to work to the advantage of millions.

Over the same years that military experience was expanding and confirming this view of disease as preventable as well as curable, civilian governments and industry were embracing a similar interpretation of disease. The budget for the state health work of North Carolina in 1909 was

$2,500; in 1921 it was $900,000. The extraordinary growth of expenditures for the public health has gone far toward losing its impressiveness because we in the Western Hemisphere see it all about us. We take it for granted. But one visit to the Orient awakens most travelers to the value of the protection afforded human happiness and life itself by the application of medical science. And one of the most reassuring aspects of public health work in the United States is that it is so largely administered by local authorities— state, county, and city.

In broad terms, I think it is probably true to say that with the exception of support for the cure of tuberculosis and mental disease, the expenditures of counties and states have been mainly in the field of preventive medicine. Industrial medicine, starting with the treatment of accidents, minor infections, and ambulatory illness and the installation of safety devices, has only of late begun to expand into the fields of general medical care and the control or prevention of disease in the mass. But both civil authorities and industrial management have this in common: they regard disease with matter-of-fact impatience, with scientific detachment, as a condition ranging from being a nuisance to being a culpable tragedy, and they regard health as a state ranging from being a demonstrable economy to being a civic right.

One still more recent change is observable relating to the current interpretation of disease. Quite significantly, our phraseology, which previously involved the word "disease," has begun to change, and we hear of health maintenance, health protection, and the health professions. This change signifies a larger horizon, a larger task, a larger number and variety of skills and personnel, but it also aims at a more positive and desirable goal than the mere absence of disease.

38   *What is the meaning of disease?*

Now that the unions are beginning to press for health protection and medical care as a part of workers' recompense, to be used for prepayment insurance, we face the nearly complete emergence of an attitude which is so different from the earlier animistic and religious concepts of disease as to call for careful reflection and continuing attention. Disease is now taken as a loss of health and strength, a loss whose likelihood is calculable for large numbers and thus adaptable to insurance procedures, a loss that can be either prevented, alleviated, or cured, and at least shared financially, and each of these activities can now be pursued with such a degree of efficiency as to justify concerted and continuous action.

What the next turning point of our understanding of disease may be is a matter for surmise and speculation. I would hazard the guess that the next interpretation of disease will in some way involve an increased emphasis on the ecological approach. Ecology is the branch of biology which deals with the mutual relations between organisms and their environment. The more we learn about living creatures, whether plant or animal, the more impressive becomes the evidence of the interrelatedness of living things. They obviously live on each other as predators or as parasites. Somewhat less obviously, they live with each other in varying degrees of mutual aid and dependence. For all its complexity, ecology provides a fascinating kind of understanding of what goes on. Paul B. Sears's paper "Human Ecology: A Problem in Synthesis,"[2] Marston Bates's book, *The Nature of Natural History*,[3] and Fraser Darling's book,

[2] Paul B. Sears, "Human Ecology: A Problem in Synthesis," *Science*, Dec. 10, 1954, Vol. 120, No. 3128, pp. 959–63.

[3] Marston Bates, *The Nature of Natural History* (New York, Charles Scribner's Sons, 1950).

A Herd of Red Deer,⁴ would reward almost any reader who wants to get an idea of what ecology means.

As a trivial but lively example of ecological thinking, there is the answer to the question, "Why would honey be abundant after devastating wars?" The argument runs as follows: After many men have been killed, there are an unusual number of widows and spinsters. Women who live alone like to keep cats. An increased number of cats which kill field mice reduces the population of field mice. Since field mice kill bumble bees, fewer field mice means more bumble bees. Bumble bees pollinate clover, thus increasing the quantity of clover, which provides more honey for honeybees.

Perhaps one of the first powerful results of interpreting disease as an ecologist would regard it would be a greater interest in convalescence and rehabilitation. Surely, it is no loss to medicine if the ecologist joins hands with the economist and the humanist in holding that the return to wage earning and independence forms part of the cure. Indeed, we are beginning to see rehabilitation as a growing fringe of Great Medicine.

In reviewing these variant interpretations that have been put upon the existence of disease, I did not stop to emphasize the fact that all these interpretations were influenced by, as well as influencing, the growth of medical knowledge. For example, it was a good deal easier to accept the interpretation that the pain of childbirth was ordained by God as woman's lot as long as there was no known chemical to alleviate such suffering. But when chloroform came to hand

⁴ F. Fraser Darling, *A Herd of Red Deer* (London, Oxford University Press, 1937).

as an alternative, the theologians very naturally clung to interpreting to the laity what they believed was God's view of the matter, while obstetricians, midwives, and expectant mothers moved, despite clerical protest, to a new interpretation of that kind of suffering, i.e., that it was unnecessary and indefensible.

May it not occasionally give us pause to reflect that in countries where the traditional religious and philosophical beliefs have all but completely reconciled the people to their lot, we bring a peculiar strain when our drugs and our technology suggest that an alternative to suffering exists . . . even though for want of foreign exchange they cannot have it? I argue here for nothing but reflectiveness. The very successes of medical science, especially in the past eight decades, have put earlier interpretations of disease to such stubborn challenge and such shattering tests that we are, without realizing it, in a new world.

Then why are we so slow to realize the value of modern medicine? Why do we drag our feet so stupidly? Why do we cheat our medical students of decently paid teachers, of adequate instruction, of fair remuneration as interns and residents? Why does aid for the construction of hospitals have to be offered by the federal government in a country that spends $4,600,000,000 annually on the rugged and individual use of tobacco? Why do we complain of the cost of a medical care and protection that has doubled the life expectancy of all the babies we introduce to America? Is God's will to be seen in an infant's death but not in intelligent activity to prevent its death? Why is it taking so long to get the consumers of preventive and curative, alleviative and restorative, medical care to learn its value? Why have we not waked up to the incredible prospects and the immeasurable advantage we enjoy? It is hard to say, but I shall offer some possible, if partial, explanations—not excuses.

Science and empirical invention have provided various technologies with the means of immense progress—as examples, the telephone, the radio, the automobile, the airplane. This has been a kind of advance that, except for the medical field, has found an outlet in quite new competitive commercial enterprises. It seems to me important to note that all of these enterprises have used advertising and, by advertising, have taught the public to understand and use their services or products. The automobile, the airplane, the radio, and television have resulted in industries, in profits, and in informative advertising. I can begin to understand why the public comprehends so little of the potentialities of medicine if I recall that medical science has not usually capitalized on its advances with a huge exploitation of a large advertising staff charged with, and well paid for, keeping the demand ahead of the supply. The potentialities of comparable technical advances in medicine have not been explained or set forth in paid advertising to the general public either by individual doctors or by hospitals. Nor do I think they should advertise. Advertising is done, obviously, by drug manufacturers, but the advertising of therapeutic services, in contrast to therapeutic substances, has had to follow quite different rules, and I submit that though the course followed has been the right course, it has not brought about an understanding of medical science on the part of the general public that equals the public understanding of the capacities and potentialities of the automobile, the airplane, or the radio.

Furthermore, the use of an automobile or of television is at the daily option of the user, while the use of comparable advances in medical technology is still associated with urgent but not exactly predictable emergencies. Since we must not advertise individual medical service, we should put more emphasis on the information of the public in matters of health in order to have the current and well-proven facts available to all. The most nearly effective agents for this purpose now are the science writers, and great credit is due to them and to the newspapers and magazines that employ them.

At the risk of seeming disrespectful of the academic mind, I would point out that although doctors should refrain from advertising, I find that advertising men present one salutary contrast to the usual professorial attitude. The professor cares deeply for the accuracy and completeness of what he says or writes but bothers somewhat less as to what impression he has conveyed; the advertiser cares deeply about the impression he creates but is, I would conclude from reading advertisements, somewhat less concerned regarding the accuracy or completeness of what he says or writes. But looked at in terms of effective communication, however, the advertiser has, it seems to me, a considerable advantage over the professor.

But the lag of the laity in understanding the potentialities of medical science goes deeper than the mere matter of being inadequately informed. Indeed, there is a mistaken attitude toward disease which I might well have mentioned earlier, but I have reserved it till now, the better to deal with it. This mistaken attitude, briefly said, is simply that accidents and illnesses are interpreted as the results, almost completely, or completely, of *chance*. Now, half-truths die hardest, and this concept of chance as deciding the incidence of disease is just such a half-truth. How often have

What is the meaning of disease? 43

you heard someone say, "Fortunately, I have enjoyed good health all my life"? How dangerously stupid is such a remark! Of any representative collection of adults I would estimate that at least 75 percent owe their being alive, and their being healthy enough to endure a lecture, not to an unbroken series of good luck alone but to the use at one time or another in their lives of money and intelligence in preventive measures taken in their behalf (but without their knowledge), or of medical or surgical diagnosis and treatment.

To consider that chance best explains the incidence, the severity, and the results of disease leads to a spurious sort of fatalism. Such fatalism expends no strength and plans no conquests. Now, it is by no mere chance that our food, our milk, and our water are safe. First came the pioneer work in bacteriology that proved the possibility of serious diseases being distributed by food or milk or water. Then came the often-obstructed efforts of hygienists and sanitarians to apply their knowledge in your behalf and mine. And then began the long chain of faithful and zealous supervisors of markets, dairies, and watersheds to whose efforts we must ascribe the safety for our casual assumption that tomorrow not in New York nor its suburbs nor in any vastly populated area in the United States shall we enter the long hell of typhoid, amebic dysentery, tuberculosis, septic sore throats, or some other avoidable infection. To think of disease in general as mere bad luck begs the question, masks the issue, and in general clouds the concept of disease by ignoring the rôle of brains and money in avoiding or curing it. Are you willing to ascribe mistakes of ignorance of an inadequately trained doctor to bad luck? No, you took no share in supplying him with a decent medical education

44 *What is the meaning of disease?*

—that is nearer the reason. True, in those diseases whose cause or convergent causes are still completely unknown it is reasonable, for want of adequate knowledge, to speak of luck or chance as being implicated. But in diseases whose cause is clearly understood, and especially where measures have already been shown to be effective, we gain nothing and lose much by speaking of disease as though it were a matter of chance. Any phenomenon, except some in the field, of physics or chemistry, that is ascribed to chance is likely to be no more understood tomorrow than it was yesterday. So, in so far as the laity ascribes disease to bad luck, they postpone understanding it.

One further fact accounts for delay in the application of the benefits of medicine to human life. And here the blame —if it be blame—falls on us doctors. We compromise too much. We live up too often only to what is expected of us and not quite often enough to what we could expect of ourselves. We are often expected to relieve pain; but we know we should look for its cause as well. The doctor's dilemma is whether to do only what the patient wants and expects or to go far beyond that often paltry, temporary, cheap, and ignorant demand and reach a fundamental, permanent, even expensive, but intelligent solution of the patient's need. In the light of what we know medicine could do, we accept too often the world as it is, forgetting that the more precise and dependable our medical science becomes, the more certainly our methods will produce results: then by just so much is our responsibility increased for producing those results.

The ease with which we incline to compromise is obviously influenced by the patient's purse; but it is also, I think, influenced by our own educational experience.

What is the meaning of disease?

Whereas a young engineer early in his training learns the properties of new and perfect structural materials and has as his task the creation of a bridge or a building more than adequate to the strains imposed on it, a medical student absorbs, usually, a quite different attitude. His first patients often possess bodily machinery that is worn or damaged. They come to him late, often too late. To that serious fact he must adjust himself. More often than not the doctor must compromise with his patient's poverty, or ignorance, or age, or weakness of character. And from the repeated exposure and attrition of constant compromise, the doctor begins to lose whatever impatient creativeness he may have had, whatever restless insistence on starting with the best material obtainable. So frequently does the doctor accept *what is*, that progress in *what might be* has come, on many an occasion, not from the resignation of the doctor but from the fresh energies of the layman who asks the doctor that liveliest of all questions, "Why not?" So great has our professional experience been with compromise and improvising that I have sometimes wondered if the letters M.D. don't stand for "Make Do." Despite recurrent waves of frustration or self-pity, let us doctors remind ourselves that some of the laggard pace in the progress of medicine cannot be ascribed to persons outside our own ranks.

What, for example, is the sense of doctors carrying on an extensive physical examination of young men when they come of military age and then looking at each other with long faces because of the number of physical defects that could have been prevented by remedial care six or twelve years before? If the state insists that children be educated beginning at the age of six so that the electorate of a democracy will be at least largely literate, why not insist, if the state is going to draft young men for military service at eighteen, that physical adequacy be encouraged from six years onward, when remedial measures could have some chance of success? In the light of what doctors now know, the age of eighteen is no time to discover serious physical defects that could be detected and corrected at the age of six or even twelve.

I beg you not to misunderstand me on this point: I do not advocate placing compulsive power into the hands of any of the health professions beyond the point determined by the understanding and desire of society at large. But I do urge a wider understanding by the public of what they could have, and when, and how, and at what cost. We doctors must be asked to do what we know can be done, for just as the best treatment is the treatment that finally puts the patient in command of the situation, so the best attitude for the health professions is one of service to an intelligent demand, including the task of seeing to it as far as can be that the demand be intelligent. The only reinforcement of his power that the doctor needs lies in the wisdom of the demands made upon him. We know how to do a great deal if you will only ask us. That is the burden of my favorite limerick:

> There was a young lady from Siam
> Who said to her lover named Py-Am
> "To kiss me, of course,
> You will have to use force,
> But God knows you're stronger than I am."

Now to conclude with a brief résumé. Throughout history and throughout the world today we can detect a variety of interpretations set upon the existence and the meaning of disease. The more primitive view finds in disease the evidence of malice or vengeance of hostile persons or malevolent spirits. Divine disfavor, or punishment for sin, have similarly long served as explanations of disease. The reactions have ranged from exorcism and expiation to abject remorse and the agony of the outcast bereft of hope. The Greek interpretation of disease had the glorious character of being rational and free in large measure of sin, guilt, malice, and superstitious terror. The Christian view that aid to the sufferer was an act of piety and that sufferers were the elect of God brought a most significant change to the way in which disease was regarded. It also brought into being hospitals, which have evolved slowly but surely into the most effective institutions of the present day for giving medical care. With the growth of precise and dependable knowledge, both military and civilian, and now industrial, agencies have come to regard medical care as a source of military and national strength, as an immense economy, as a form of recompense, and in certain cases as a civic right. Possibly the next major development in the interpretation of disease will stress the ecological approach—that is, the recognition of the intimate yet extensive interrelatedness of the organism and its environment, i.e., the patient and the rest of us. But in any event, what was done about disease may be shown to be closely related, if not, indeed, directly indicative, of what was taken to be the meaning of disease.

Our slowness in using medical science as it could be used is due in part to thinking that chance decides whether we shall be well or sick. It seems also to be due to the fact that medical services possess no appropriate and fully adequate means of informing and educating the public to the present potentialities of medical care, both preventive and curative. Perhaps, too, the medical profession suffers somewhat from its unceasing necessity to compromise with the patient's ideas of what he wants, what he can do, and what he can pay for. But it is of immense significance that in increasing measure what is good for the few is seen to be good for the many. The health professions must get themselves asked to do what they already know can be done.

3. Current factors affecting medicine

DURING the past thirty years I have had the unusual experience of visiting, once or repeatedly, the medical schools of some forty countries. I am perfectly aware of the fact that mere breadth or variety of experience cannot be equated with perceptiveness, or with wisdom, in interpreting the wide variety of conditions seen. But I should feel almost a sense of guilt if such a privileged experience were "lodged with me useless" and I could make no effort to share some part of the impressions received or make some statement of the inferences drawn, so that others can, if they choose, take some vicarious and partial advantage from such an accumulation of experience.

Among the residues of this experience I would record one conviction that was not at the outset not even on my horizon, but which, as I visited more and more countries, and as time for reflection increased, not only established itself in my mind but steadily grew in volume and in strength. This was the realization that in order to understand the meaning of Great Medicine in any country one must study its historical, social, cultural, economic, and scientific matrix. Within Great Medicine I mean to include the teaching, the practice, and the research in medicine, in all its roots as well as all its branches. We need some such deliberately inclusive term lest confusion arise from the fact that the word "medicine" is used in contradistinction to surgery, or it may mean what is poured from a bottle. In using the term matrix I mean the environment, the attendant circumstances, the accompanying conditions, the general surroundings of Great Medicine.

If it took years of experience to show me the importance of the historical, social, cultural, economic, and scientific matrix of Great Medicine, then two inferences are possible (but not mutually exclusive): one, that I was not quick to grasp the obvious, and the other, that this matrix, or, rather, these matrices, are more important than is usually realized. At any rate, the essential point is this: Medical research, teaching, and practice depend directly and sensitively upon many environmental factors—perhaps more immediately and completely than we have realized.

Studies of interactions, of environmental influences, of multiple variables, are notoriously elusive to make and difficult to communicate. The various kinds of environment surrounding Great Medicine are hard to present in their totality. For my present purposes, therefore, I should like to consider only some of the current circumstances affecting Great Medicine—the practice and the teaching of medicine, and the research clearly within medicine, or at least within its growing frontiers. For there are now forces in play that are strong enough and intimate enough to change the organization and methods and perhaps some, even, of the immediate objectives of medical practice, teaching, and research. It is not easy to determine or to present the interplay at any one moment of several forces that are themselves changing in character and strength. In physics one can speak of the parallelogram of forces, but the present task is infinitely more complicated. Even the more apparent of

Current factors affecting medicine 51

these factors are so numerous that although I could mention several, I could not discuss them thoroughly here.

The first factor I choose to mention is prepayment for medical care. Prepayment can be made for the costs of hospitalization exclusive of the fees for professional care, or it can be made for professional care apart from hospitalization. And, obviously, the prepayment procedure can in one way or another be made to cover hospital costs and professional care and supervision. Historically, organizations for prepayment for hospital expenses preceded, in the main, and in most countries, the development of programs or organizations employing prepayment to meet the fees of doctors or other personal professional charges. The growth and development of prepayment programs can be better understood if we remember a few of the characteristics of such plans.

Prepayment involves, of course, the principle of insurance. In the absence of precise knowledge of morbidity rates applicable in the way that dependable life tables provide a safe basis for life insurance, prepayment enterprises have protected themselves, partially at least, by insisting on taking in groups of voluntary subscribers chosen in such a way as to include a safe number of expectably well persons rather than a self-selected accumulation of probable chronic invalids. We have still so scant a knowledge of the incidence and nature of disease that the success of Blue Cross and Blue Shield has been notable, if we remember that we knew and still know very little, statistically, as to the amount of illness to be expected per 100,000 of population. I think it fair to suppose that at the outset of such programs probably more depended on caution and consistency in the administration of prepayment health insurance than on the exactitude with which contracts could be approximated to the actual incidence, severity, and duration of all kinds of disease. Indeed, one of the retarding factors in the spread of prepayment health insurance has been the caution necessary in point of coverage, especially in such diseases as tuberculosis and mental disorders and chronic diseases. Even so, the trend to sickness insurance has shown power. Why? The strength of the movement for prepayment for medical care lies in the number of persons whose individual incomes simply cannot withstand the catastrophic effect of incapacitating illness.

To say that the prepayment principle affects practitioners of medicine is a considerable understatement. Indeed, prepayment plans lie in the very area where the views of the consumers of medical care are likely to be at variance with the purveyors thereof. There are even programs in which the representation of one or the other is explicitly subordinated or even omitted. Another clear evidence of the demand for, and the already considerable effectiveness of, the prepayment principle, can be seen in the fact that some insurance companies now provide, on the basis of commercial contracts, a wide variety of coverage. The growing experience of prepayment plans makes more precise and more liberal protection increasingly likely. In other words, this is a change in medical care that has come to stay—and to grow. Its effects will be immense. How may it affect research and teaching?

From the early days of the *Krankenkassen* in central Europe and the panel system championed by Lloyd George in 1912, the more thoughtful observers have offered the criticism that the tendency of health insurance schemes has been to build more hospitals but not to be alert to the extraordinary economy of successful research or rigorous preventive measures. No one can deny that human society throughout the world owes more to universities, foundations, and private donors, and particularly to the abnegation of research workers themselves, for the progress of medical science and its immense economy in improving medical care, than to the administration, at least up to now, of prepayment health insurance plans. That is a serious criticism in the light of the certainty that the contributions of our fellow citizens to health insurance plans are likely, in the next decade, to reach a magnitude that in 1930 was unbelievable. Nor need the criticism be left to the future to prove its force. Right now there are too many hospitals that take the position that research and teaching costs should come from the university or from private donors, as though the quality of patient care had nothing to gain from the work and the presence of research men and teachers. On this palpably false assumption the universities are being mulcted of funds to pay for a level of care they could more justly be paid for providing to the hospitals. I know that no easy formula will distinguish between educational expenses and expenses of patient care. I know the hospital cost per diem is high, and mounting. I know that unexpected illness is distressingly expensive. But I also know that, since hospital care is more valuable today than it has ever been and is growing more so every year, we deceive ourselves and each other by haggling over the cost of adequate health insurance. Relative to less urgent items on our budgets, such as liquor, tobacco, cosmetics, amusements, and the fripperies, this is stupid or improvident in the extreme. The table from the Hartford Hospital demands attention. In this table it is assumed that Patient A's income was, in 1888,

$852. This corresponds to $2,500 for Patient B, in 1948. In 1888, $852 went as far as $2,500 did in 1948.

Sixty Years Difference at Hartford Hospital

	Patient A—1888	Patient B—1948
Patient-day cost	$1.09	$18.08
Length of stay	52 days	8.5 days
Cost of hospitalization	$56.68	$153.68
Yearly income	$852.00	$2,500.00
Work-day income	$2.77	$8.14
Days of work needed to pay hospital bill	20	19
Work days lost while in hospital	44	7
Total days lost	64	26
Percent of income lost	21	8.5

The effect of Blue Cross, Blue Shield, and the commercial contracts on medical education occasion surprise. In the days when a great deal of medical care was given in the name of charity by the voluntary hospitals, or as tax-supported aid to the indigent in the city and county hospitals, there were always patients in plenty available for teaching medical students, interns, and, mark you, for teaching the "professor doctor," too. Parenthetically, I might add that it was precisely the extent and length of experience with these patients that gave the "professor doctor" much of the skill and wisdom he possessed, and hence his prestige. And, conversely, it has been long since true, though not widely recognized, that the charity patients of teaching hospitals receive better diagnosis and treatment than many a private patient in a non-teaching private hospital. That may seem a disturbing statement, so I'll call your attention to the fact that I did not say that all ward patients get better treatment than all private or semi-private patients. But in the light of what I know about hospitals and human nature, the next time I am ill in a hospital I am going to go to a teaching hospital and ask (and, if strong enough at the time, insist) that I be used for teaching. It would be perhaps too strong language to say I'll do this in self-protection, but not to say that I'll do it for the cost-free advantage it might bring me. It is high time the general public understood the advantages of going to a teaching hospital, for being used for teaching invokes some additional attention given to diagnosis, treatment, and care, because all three are exposed to a far larger number of critics and questions in a teaching hospital than elsewhere. The layman does not know how to obtain this advantage. He has never realized that, in medicine, charity offers to the poor the gains in medical skill, not the leavings. The usual layman doesn't trust anything connected or associated with being poor. It is the pathetic fate of the middle class that they want appearances even more than solid value. As an example, taken from the field of automobiles, the rich man could afford the *appearance* as well as the *performance* of a Peerless. The poor man stuck to value in a Model T. The man from the middle class took a cut in performance and appearance. In point of medical care the rich can afford both value and appearances, the poor must think of value, but the middle class wanting both—which they can't afford—often prefers appearances and so loses more important things in medical care than deference, convenience, and a nice bedside manner.

And now with the advent of prepayment plans to cover the cost of medical care, the proportion of charity cases diminishes. But, far more significant, the immense contribution of the charity patients to medical education has begun to disappear. Let us imagine an example. In 1910 a cabdriver suffering from gallstones consulted a private practitioner not on the staff of the local medical school or its hospital. The patient had no savings, and it was before the days of Blue Cross or Blue Shield. Who was there to pay for adequate care? The practitioner could only say, "Go to the Presbyterian Hospital: they'll take care of you." So the patient went, and was used for teaching, and at the operation two or three young surgeons in training had the experience of assisting at or doing a gall bladder operation. If today a similar patient with Blue Cross and Blue Shield membership consults his practitioner, he is likely to be told, "I'll be glad to get you into the X-Y-Z hospital and operate on you myself next Tuesday." Consequently, the medical schools and the interns and the residents and even the professors of surgery in the charity and city hospitals are feeling the loss of adequate experience because of a decline in the number of patients who enter the hospital as charity patients.

Another major development affecting Great Medicine today is the growth of specialism. It affects practice, teaching, and research, especially in the countries that are thickly settled or well supplied with automobiles, and where the population possesses on the average a relatively large amount of information and money. These attendant circumstances being true of the United States, or of many parts of it, one cannot be surprised at the growth here of specialism in all the forms of medical care. And in the popular interpretation of the specialists we have another example of the significance of an attitude. Robert Lynd, a sociologist at Columbia University, shrewdly pointed out in a talk he gave at the New York Academy of Medicine that although forty years ago the death of a small child was likely to cause some such comment as "Isn't it too bad that God has called for that small boy!" the commoner comment today would be "Why didn't they call a specialist earlier?" Whenever neighbors' comment moves from an exclamation point to a question mark, conditions are beginning to change.

Though I would not expect specialists to flourish and multiply where the roads are bad, the population sparse, the people poor and ignorant, I would not deny that another and quite different reason has affected the growth of specialism. This is the immense advance and accumulation of useful knowledge. This continues. But, as in most other examples of growth, what determines the value and advantage of growth is the excellence of the accompanying organization, coordination, and communication. What is the advantage of a huge city without streets and without government? Looking at the whole field of health services and medical care, one can now count some thirty or more professional careers that call for special instruction and coordination. Mere recital will serve to convince you. Starting with the familiar family physician or general practitioner, we have: internists, surgeons, pediatricians, obstetricians and gynecologists, pathologists, radiologists, neurologists, psychiatrists, clinical psychologists, orthopedists, urologists, ophthalmologists, dermatologists, physiotherapists, occupational therapists, corrective therapists, nurses, attendants, hospital administrators, public health officers, industrial physicians, military medical officers of at least three categories (air, sea, and land), biometricians, biochemists, and a good many more if you count many of the surgical and medical specialties—neurosurgeons, phthisiologists, cardiologists, allergists, proctologists, and anesthesiologists. Nor does this list include teachers of some ten special subjects, like anatomy, physiology, bacteriology, pathology, pharmacology, and others, whose work underlies the work of the clinical men and leads it forward.

The task of coordination or effective collaboration of so many specialties gives us all pause. Indeed, when you realize that each of these specialties calls for special training lasting from one to five years or more; that many of the specialists depend on each other's services and must learn to collaborate, and must keep up to date in their own work; and that most of them have national associations, with officers to elect, and many have examinations to conduct for membership, and conventions to attend, and papers to prepare, and occasional surveys to find out how they are doing, such goals as adequate coordination of the specialist's work with that of others prove extraordinarily difficult for the conscientious specialist.

The more serious fact about the specialties seems to me to be this: The training necessary to produce a competent specialist in the medical profession now takes three to five years subsequent to acquiring the M.D. degree. Whereas Abraham Flexner attacked the forms that medical education followed in 1910 because the latter part of the then four-year course was in the hands of men who were primarily practitioners and only secondarily teachers, a similar situation again confronts medical education, whose latter half is now devoted in many instances to meeting the requirements not of universities, but of the specialty boards. Indeed, only the schools of public health provide, under university auspices and with any considerable fraction of full-time teachers, a course of graduate training directly comparable to the course required for the M.D. degree.

I do not believe that the total effect of the specialty boards has been bad, certainly not if their purpose has been to force up the average level of all specialists by holding to a minimum standard. But the capacity to pass written and oral examinations is just that and not always more. The examiner does not find out what the candidate knows; he only finds out whether the candidate knows what the examiner knows. In stagnant fields the old know more than the young, and then certification by examination makes sense. The paradox of specialty board certification is that it hurries a process in which preeminence and maturity should be the major considerations. You don't find preeminence by setting minimal standards, and you don't encourage maturity by rewarding the precocious. The danger is that the originality and freedom to go beyond the knowledge of older practitioners is not adequately encouraged. I would more gladly see the task of selecting and rewarding originality and mature competence entrusted to full-time teachers and investigators than to practitioners. I suspect that the specialty boards have grown in power and influence more because our medical schools are weakening and are now unable to undertake the burden of training specialists than because the capacity to pass written and oral examinations is the ideal objective of research or really advanced teaching.

The most nearly satisfactory practical corrective of the defects of specialism is group practice. More than one reason supports such an opinion, though in other countries than the United States group practice has made but little headway. First, the skills as well as the knowledge in all the fields of Great Medicine exceed, by an indisputable margin, the abilities of any one man to master. Secondly, it is possible for professional men to collaborate effectively in the care of any patient. Thirdly, group practice encourages, facilitates, and improves such collaboration, and to the advantage of the patient. Thus far the argument is self-evident and familiar.

There are, also, less evident advantages. Perhaps these can best be brought out by the sarcastic remark I once heard that there's very little difference between group practice and fee-splitting unless the performance of every member of the group is held to a high level. In other words, the service given a patient by group practice gains in quality by the criticism of the other members of the group, whether the criticism be tacit or fully expressed. Whether we realize it or not, the presence of merely a competent trained nurse tends to raise the doctor's level of performance. Reluctant as an anxious patient may be to think that his doctor, above all people, might ever need the stimulus of competent critics, the fact remains that doctors sometimes do need, and usually respond well, to the realization that their work is observable and observed. Usually no more than that is needed, but if censure is needed and yet not forthcoming, then the group clinic is not much stronger than its weakest link and usually is in need of reorganization.

The similarity between group practice and practice in a well-organized teaching hospital with full-time staff has had two results, as I see it. The first is that the transition to group practice from working in a good teaching hospital as a student, intern, resident, or young instructor proves to be fraught with fewer risks and difficulties than going into practice alone. Thus one could say that group practice is growing because medical education under full-time teachers prepares a young man almost specifically for group practice.

The other results of the similarity between group practice and full-time clinical units is the question that is now being raised as to whether faculties of medicine should not be organized as group practices. Here I might point out one of the attractions of group practice: Income taxes are now so high that overworking to produce a large net income in private practice appeals less than it did, and the retirement arrangements, vacations, and coverage during illness or absence that characterize many group practice positions, together with reasonable but dependable salaries, make group practice worth the consideration of many men who would not have gone into it before the income tax laid so heavy a hand on the doctor's gross and net income.

There are, however, two dissimilarities between group practice and a faculty of medicine. Both of these dissimilarities argue against organizing schools of medicine around the structure of group practice. In the first place, group practice centers logically and appropriately around the care of the patient and little else, whereas the task of a clinician in a teaching hospital involves two additional duties—teaching and research. If a member of a group practice doesn't handle patients ingratiatingly and do his work well as a practitioner, then his departure from the group is due on logical as well as psychological grounds. But a member of a medical faculty may be gifted as an investigator or as a teacher but not particularly deft at handling patients, and yet be convinced of his competence in just that point. To dismiss him from his professorship would be a mistake for quite other reasons than the affront he would take it to be: a valuable teacher or investigator would be lost, which is serious for a faculty but perhaps less so for a group clinic. Secondly, if for financial reasons (and I have heard of no others) a clinical faculty were to be organized as a group practice, appointments to the faculty could not be expected to overlook the candidate's ability as a money-maker. That type of man is not unfamiliar; nearly every medical school I know has one or more on the clinical faculty, to the sorrow and disappointment as well as occasionally to the envy of his academic colleagues and the virginal awe of the students.

By and large, I could think of no more deceptively destructive device for throwing away the best potentialities of full time medical education than organizing medical faculties on the basis of group practice. Furthermore, to organize a medical faculty into a form of group practice invites the opposition as well as the jealousy of the practitioners in the community who are not on the faculty. To minimize any misunderstanding, we might add that a substantial increase of group clinics would improve the practice of medicine, and especially surgery, very appreciably. So it is no reflection on group practice to say that its essentials are not the essentials of teaching or research.

Another force impinging on the practice and teaching of medicine and, in a special way, on research, may be seen in the growth and importance of what are perhaps too condescendingly described as the ancillary services. Since effective collaboration between human beings depends first of all, and last of all, on their characters and qualities, I can hope for very little from mere semantic devices, titular upgrading, or attempting to effect actual harmony among human beings merely by making organization charts and hierarchical definitions. The respect of subordinates, like the consent of the governed, controls the quality of authority and the effectiveness of leaders in teamwork.

If we had an adequate number of these paramedical coworkers right now, the effectiveness of physicians, surgeons, public health officers, and all comparable professional personnel would be remarkably multiplied. The need to train nurses in America today is distressing. To meet the existent need for trained nurses in military and civilian life would require four out of every ten girls in our graduating high school classes for some four or five years. Since six out of every ten marry within three years of graduation and since other occupations now compete with nursing, the requisite numbers of young girls to look after their brothers in military service are not being found. If the rationale of selective service were applied to the drafting of girls of eighteen for two years of civilian nursing to match the military service of their brothers, we would create a notable and valuable reserve of nurses in this country for years to come, as well as a chance to open wards in our civilian hospitals now empty for the lack of nurses. I do not find any cogent arguments against such a resolution of the present immense problem of nursing care; the psychological resistance and the emotional resentment would be real, but just what do young women do in return for citizenship? And would not most of the future activities of young women of eighteen be done better if more had a nurse's training?

Among the changes during the past century in what hospitals are and in what they do, the trend toward specialization is obvious. One could almost say that instead of being the place where a doctor could easily see a great many kinds of patients, the hospital has become the place where a patient can see a great many kinds of doctors. The change is radical but it is not simple. In a large modern hospital one finds not only a great variety of specialists, all members of the medical profession, but also a great many specialists who are not doctors but whose knowledge, skills, and work provide indispensable services to the patients. It may surprise you to know that hospital managers have listed 180 such subdivisions of service rendered directly or indirectly in the care of the hospital patient, to mention only a few: trained nurses, supervisors, nurses aides, male nurses and attendants, physiotherapists, social workers, nutritionists, dentists, hospital administrators. Many of these categories need special training of upwards of a year, and, once trained, such specialists occupy an acknowledged position in the total personnel of the hospital, with well-defined responsibilities. How far specialization may sensibly be pushed, or even allowed, depends on the amount of work to be done. Very naturally, the larger the hospital the larger the number of persons who may need, for example, the attention of a nutritionist.

We do not pay quite enough attention to the fact that many of such special skills or services are represented, but each by only one person in the hospital. Since she is alone, any wide fluctuation in the demand for her services will create difficulty, and much—perhaps too much—depends upon her personal characteristics, particularly her capacity to resist self-pity and resentment at not being understood, or appreciated, or "given a chance." As specialization increases, the need for coordination of the different skills becomes more acute—coordination not merely in purely administrative terms but the kind of coordination that comes from mutual understanding, effective communications, and teamwork.

Just as the business schools have discovered that the art of personnel management, industrial psychology, and the like deserve and reward emphatic attention, so instructors in the medical specialties, both professional and nonprofessional, should give explicit attention to personnel management.

At the base of the study of management you will find the problem of authority. Not only are there different concepts of the true nature of authority, the differences can give rise to serious trouble. If professional nursing first saw the light of day—or at least the light of Florence Nightingale's lamp —when the Victorian assumptions of masculine superiority and of the military theory of command were undisputed in a highly stratified society, then some growing pains were in store for nursing in a democracy, together with headaches for those who still postpone their study of the real nature of authority and how it relates to the effective management of human beings. I think that medical students and interns need particularly to reflect upon and learn the essentials of management and the importance of the consent of the governed in any sort of government. Success will but rarely attend the assumption that effective collaboration derives primarily from organization charts or stipulated chains of command, subordination, and hierarchies. The primary source is quite different—and painfully beyond the pride or the intelligence of many administrators. Names, ranks, titles, and the like do not, in my experience, offer a solution or a preventive to what happens when, for example, a second-rate human being is put above a superior one. We need a deal of study and action if we are to see anything but prolonged friction and frustration come out of the growing complications of increasingly diversified groups in the medical and health fields.

Related to the multiplication of specialties is the increased length of medical education. The relationship is one of interaction: neither is exclusively the cause or merely the effect of the other. Looking back even fifty years, particularly in North America, one can see that the lead in lengthening the course of medical studies was taken by the schools that were accorded leadership on other counts. From two years the period of medical studies grew to four. An extra year or more of internship at first gained quiet approval, then open encouragement, and then the status of a requirement, if not for obtaining a license to practice, then at least as one of the prerequisites for certification by any specialty board. Even our military services, though hard pressed for medical officers, strongly prefer men who have had at least one year of internship. To the internship following medical school has been added one or, commonly, two or even four years of further experience in what are called residencies. The time one can assume as desirable for a thorough medical education stands, therefore, between six and nine years after graduation from college. No one needs to be told that from every point of view, except that of the consumer of the young doctor's services, that is a long time. Nor can there be much doubt that the consumer's viewpoint deserves consideration. In other words, if young doctors can manage to hold on through so long a period of preparation, what good reason can there be for preventing them?

Certainly one factor in this lengthening of medical education in this country deserves serious consideration. In lengthening the preparation for the practice of medicine by two years of obligatory military medical service we may price ourselves out of the market of well-qualified young men. A high school student in the course of choosing a career learns that preparation for medicine calls for a minimum of ten years more of education and economic dependency, or if he is to get the best of medical education even sixteen years, after graduating from high school before he can earn his living when and where he pleases. Can we blame him if he reluctantly decides to forego such a career? Such decisions do not get into statistics I have seen. The situation may appeal as an investment but hardly otherwise—and investments are supposed to pay off. Who can expect young doctors to remain free of concern for dollars and cents, if only to pay back what they have borrowed?

It is not an answer to say that more students apply for entrance to medical school than are admitted. One needs only to remember the Greeks' observation that only two groups in society can kill human beings with impunity: judges and doctors. This observation points to some emphasis upon the quality we can rightly require of medical students as well as upon the number.

I hold this lengthening of medical education to be so important that I shall devote the last lecture in this series to what I have called, "The Natural History of the Doctor," though I would call your attention now to still another force now having a powerful effect in lengthening the training period.

Under currently effective legislation, doctors are being drafted for two years of military service. The most obvious effect of this law is its lengthening of the period before a young doctor can start his own practice. This revision means that after three or four years of college come certainly four years of medical school, almost certainly one year of internship, then two years of military service, and then one to five years of residencies. Counting the premedical preparation in college, the prospect ranges from at least ten up to sixteen years of training before a young doctor can start practice. I could name from among the generation of my teachers doctors who had no college education and only three years in medical school with no subsequent internship before starting to practice—three years after high school in contrast to ten or sixteen. And since such a lengthening of medical training may give rise to queries as to whether it is now too long, I would say that the quality of professional competence in the over-all treatment and prevention of disease among North Americans has benefited in comparable measure to this lengthening of training.

One more among the many consequences of the present military situation impinges on American medicine. We are adding veterans at the rate of 30,000 to 46,000 a month—veterans returning to civilian life after a fairly impressive experience of medical care given at government expense. They then join for the rest of their lives the ranks of those eligible for care by the Veterans Administration. With some 22,000,000 of the electorate now eligible for Veterans Administration medical care, and not without ways to express themselves politically about it, I see in this situation a powerful force pushing for wider and more explicit acceptance of medical care maintained by taxation rather than as a boon given to the poor in the name of charity or purchased by the rich or even prudently assured through prepayment on the voluntary insurance basis.

The real competition will come, it seems to me, not between private practice and socialized medicine but between voluntary prepayment plans and socialized medicine. I speak of the bulk of medical practice, for private practice will continue, as private schools and colleges have continued despite the competition of socialized education, more

Current factors affecting medicine

commonly referred to as our glorious American public school system. Moreover, private practice will continue, and hospitals for private practitioners and private patients will continue, for reasons comparable to the reasons that keep private schools, colleges, and charities alive and, as I think, invaluable. But the ranks of the veterans continue to increase, and at least 22,000,000 are moving onward to their less robust and more dependent years while no one, no group, nor any political party appears eager to deal candidly with the question of care for veterans' non-service-connected disabilities. For the bulk of the population, however, the issue is going to be much more nearly between voluntary prepayment plans and some form of government-supported medical care, whether through taxation or compulsory prepayment, than between private practice and government-supported medical care. Note that the viewpoint, the facilities, and the number of our medical schools represent the past prevalence of private practice and not the needs of the population as they would show in a system of government-supported care.

I believe voluntary prepayment preferable to any other method because it avoids centralized bureaucratic control, insures variety, comparison, and adaptability of plans, and facilitates experiment and initiative, and particularly because voluntary insurance stimulates the vigilance that is the price of freedom and so educates the consumers of medical care. Again, the analogy to our public schools is not very remote. By placing responsibility for our public schools as closely as possible on the immediate users and not on the federal government or even to any very serious degree on the state government, we educate the local school boards and the parent-teacher associations—indeed, all concerned—and leave the door open to freedom, variety, and progress.

Still another immensely powerful factor in Great Medicine today is research. I shall not belabor the obvious fact that its results have gone beyond the imagination even of those prophets who in the past fifty years could have claimed serious attention. Any adequate listing of the triumphs of research in medical science would soon exhaust the very sensibility and discrimination I would prefer to preserve, just as an orchestra playing too long at fortissimo would turn excitement into insult and all sense of contrast into an intolerable monotony. Let me instead refer to a few aspects of research that have interested me.

Research is like roulette. The bank, or the house, is society with its body of established knowledge, and over the long run the house will win. A single turn of the wheel, a single research project, may win nothing. But the house's apparently small advantage brings the aggregate of many gambles to certain profit. Finding a first-class mind that happens to be at work on a good lead has an element of chance in and of itself, for chance, as Pasteur said, favors the prepared mind. And like roulette, research, as a gamble, pays off at times with a bountifulness that is almost intoxicating. Since chance, as has long been observed, has neither memory nor conscience, you can't count on research to be conscientiously responsive or otherwise mindful of the fact that you've been putting down money on research now for quite a while. Lady Luck never feels obliged to smile. That is why no honest research man will promise success on any stipulated number of projects or experiments. Indeed, the best research men I've known are so passionately skeptical

Current factors affecting medicine 71

of mere hopefulness, and yet so incurably hopeful, that it is extremely easy to mistake their almost truculent honesty, or their agonized modesty, for neurotic timidity or blunt pessimism—and yet not quite that, for, rightly, they keep at their research.

There is certain evidence in the history of research for the belief that some discoveries could not have been made until some other discovery had been made. This fact underlies an aspect of research that has nothing to do with our roulette or chance. But it does have to do with the imagination and creativeness of a good researcher. It underlies, too, what are called "good leads," for when knowledge in one field reaches a given stage, men in other fields may see how to incorporate that new knowledge or method in fruitful ways. And sometimes they may not: witness the lapse of time between the synthesis of one of the sulfa drugs in 1908 and its successful use in bacterial infections in the thirties. This dependence of some discoveries on antecedent discoveries furnishes the main reason for saying, "You can't just go out and buy the discoveries you want." Some discoveries have cost a good deal of money. But one can't infer from that fact that spending a good deal of money will buy whatever you want. In Professor V. R. Khanolkar's laboratory in Bombay I saw an excellent statement: *"Il faut chercher pour trouver mais pas pour trouver ce qu'on cherche"*—you must search to find but not to find what you are searching for.

The fantastic economies of successful research swiftly go beyond any method of accurate accounting. As an example, I would estimate that the work on the sulfa drugs up to and including the proof of their efficiency in the treatment of lobar pneumonia did not cost more than $150,000. But in as short a time as three years after their value in pneumonia was shown, the saving in life insurance policies that would have been paid by one life insurance company for deaths from lobar pneumonia alone only on the West Coast of the United States, over only one year, was calculated at $3,000,000. In such ways research gives a continuing and a permanent lift to Great Medicine.

One drawback of the present popular confidence in research is that the donors of research funds have overlooked or underestimated the importance of the medical education that will provide an adequate supply of good researchers in the future. The donors have also ignored the importance of giving first-rate research men today the salaries and tenure they deserve. As between donor and recipient, the relationship, especially in short-term grants, suggests a grim variant of the declaration that it is more blessed to give than to receive—it is certainly more comfortable. For the plain fact of the matter is that most of our medical schools often find that the full cost of research is not covered by the grants which are supposed to pay for it. The schools cannot afford any longer to accept the full moral responsibility, but only part of the full cost, of many research projects.

Other impacts of research on medical education have become increasingly powerful and evident in the past twenty years. Both for teachers and students the process of acquiring new facts in a way that is critical and discriminating has taken the place of the process of acquiring merely a selection of static facts well arranged for memorization. The full-time teacher has become more and more nearly the only one who can keep up with the constant flow of new knowledge. I know a good many such full-time teachers who are not only candid but emphatic in saying that they are not able to keep up. The pressure increases for the professor to delegate, compartmentalize, and thus to contribute to the more serious faults of specialization. As a reaction, there is a great deal of talk about integration, but it seems frequently asked of the student but never exemplified in the person of a teacher—another factor in the students' trend toward early specialization. The more conscientious graduate of ten or more years ago either wants to catch up by means of refresher courses, or he does what he can to keep up his reading, or he decides to practice medicine as he learned it and rely on the agents of the pharmaceutical companies and other agents of supply houses to give him the highlights on the new drugs. The range of the doctor's human reaction to this state of affairs is very wide; one can only envy the possessor of such natural equanimity, heroic physique, and quick intelligence under circumstances that call for all three. For a conscientious private practitioner, the changing character of what he is expected to know "all about," and be able to do, produces, I suspect, a tension that goes far to explain his intolerance as well as his anxiety at the prospect of socialized medicine. He is too harried to be calm. He is likely to resent the problems of adjusting to those whom he can deal with more easily as plain employees or at least unquestioning subordinates than as critical collaborators conscious of their newly acquired status.

A further factor affecting all aspects of Great Medicine today is inflation. It has sent the cost of medical education steadily and seriously upward, especially since 1945. Coming on top of the dislocations of the war and the spuriously prosperous income of the speed-up in taking in war-time classes in rapid succession, inflation has added further injury to schools whose endowment income had been already cut by a third during the depression. The cumulative effect of all these difficulties was discernible in 1947. It has been unrelenting ever since and now is all but disastrous.

For some reason or reasons I do not understand, the American medical schools have not taken their case effectively to the general public. Organized medicine has opposed recourse to government aid. At the initiative of a few of the leading university presidents, an organization was formed in 1950 to attempt to secure from lay sources an adequate increase of income for medical education. However, the results of this effort have not been impressive as yet. Numerous reports of the problems of the medical schools' financial status are available, whose thoroughness does not find a proportionately prompt or adequate response. I think the situation serious.

Following the accepted practice in hospitals when patients become dangerously ill, American medical education should be put on the Dangerous List. That practice is simply a formal notification from the hospital authorities, who could be held responsible, to the patient's relatives, who can be assumed to be interested. It is a direct and unmistakable notice that all is far from being well. Without such notice the relatives could very justly complain that they should have been told that the patient was dangerously ill. It seems clear to me that the American public has a legitimate, indeed, an indisputable, stake and interest in the work of the medical schools. If the Association of American Medical Colleges delays or refuses to tell the public that the work of training doctors is faltering and, indeed, deteriorating for the lack of support, then that Association evades its moral duty. Furthermore, the medical profession, the richest profession in point of average earned income per member, cuts a poor figure as a beggar to laymen when its members received at least one third and often two thirds of the costs of their medical education without paying while in school or later. If each doctor now in practice would send back to his medical school $100 a year, we should have $20,000,000 yearly for medical education instead of the pitiable response thus far obtained by the National Fund for Medical Education. And each doctor could send $100 for each of twenty years without repaying for what has been given him.

As a reluctant witness of the present deterioration in American medical education and of the threat of the still worse deterioration in store, I warn you in tones that are neither shrill nor strident that the members of the medical profession should begin to pay back what they received from endowments, gifts, and public taxation and that laymen should be made aware, too, of the price they will pay if medical schools cannot train doctors as they know how to train them. As an old Frenchman said to a friend of mine, "Remember, my boy, you can have anything you want in this world, but don't forget to pay for it."

As I have indicated, the teaching, research, and practice of medicine are changing under the influence of a number of facts and forces. So intimately do research, teaching, and practice act and interact on each other that any factor that may seem to modify only one actually affects the others. Inflation, for example, swiftly changes medical education, and in so doing reduces the number of competent younger research workers and in many instances makes the medical school play the white elephant in the budget of an impoverished university.

In medical education the chief adverse forces are inflation, the present scarcity of patients as a result of prepayment plans, the scarcity of students in the paramedical professions, such as nursing, and the growth of specialism. But I see none of these as insuperable if the medical profession will adequately inform the laity of the present state of affairs and of the results that will follow if nothing is done.

In research the limiting factors seem to me to come from a lack of understanding of research on the part of governments, foundations, and personal supporters. They do not understand the nature of research or the way of the investigator. Consequently, grants in which the donor hides his ignorance under the cloak of caution have become common, and in the absence of steadfast support the stage is set, or rather the audience is primed, for the quick, the easily described, and the applicable additions to knowledge. Nonetheless, with a thousand examples of waste and waywardness, medical research will continue.

In the practice of medicine economic, social, cultural, and political factors have produced an exceedingly complicated condition. It seems to me that the essential elements are the growing general appreciation of the value of medical care regardless of how it is paid for, an increasing probability that medical care will be most effectively organized and paid for on the basis of prepayment insurance, and an increasing attention to the psychological as well as the economic aspects of hospital and other forms of administration of medical care. As a final observation, this might be added: the costs of medical education will at long last be found to be only a part of the costs of medical care, because medical education will have to be a preparation to meet not merely the demand but the need for medical care.

4. How are medical education and medical care best paid for?

THE appropriate time has come for a restatement of the themes of the previous chapters. This I would offer you now not as a review or summation or reiteration but in the hope that by using somewhat different terms and language, statements that were too brief or not quite clear can take on their proper significance in your minds.

When we stop to think how much more effectively the medical practitioner, and all the helpers he calls upon, can deal with disease today than he could a hundred years ago, the contrast deserves a greater compliment than wonder or applause. It deserves sober reflection and study, even to the point of raising the question "Do we fully realize how remarkably valuable Great Medicine has become?" When we study the detailed and credible evidence of what medical science and practical skill have come to offer over the past three generations, and especially within memories of living men today, we can very fairly ask the ironic question "How dear is life?" I say "ironic question," since on all sides, as it seems, there is reluctance to pay for dear life simply because we have come to take it for granted. We are lulled into a sort of apathy by our protection from, or survival of, diseases that would long since have decimated our population had medical science remained unchanged since 1856. Decimation originally meant the killing of one in ten, but far more than one in ten of my readers would be dead or too frail to endure an evening of reading had not medical protection and medical care benefited them sometime, or many times, in their past.

I plead with you to exercise some measure of historical sense, for only so can you realize that it is nearer 90 percent than 10 percent of you who are alive and in your present state of health, thanks to the application of medical science. Further reflection would make it more than evident that in more instances than you realize your health has remained good because of the protection now afforded you, through safe water, clean milk, the protection that inoculations give against such diseases as typhoid, tetanus, and diphtheria, and the control of mosquitoes carrying the malaria that in the past hundred years was common enough in the United States. You would, furthermore, agree that advances in the scientific knowledge of nutrition have become commonplace knowledge of millions of housewives, to the immense advantage of growing children, working adults, and active old folks—now, I am told, to be called persons of "advanced maturity." And in addition to such a list, you can contemplate, in terms of comfort as well as survival, what it means to be able to rely on surgical operations, which anesthesia robs of the terror of pain and asepsis robs of the old-time horror of gangrene or long-term suppuration. If you seek a lively sense of progress in medicine, let me remind you that pus used to be called "God's salve." The sulfa drugs and particularly the antibiotics have removed most of the danger of mastoid infections, pneumonia, and venereal disease. And still you say that *fortunately* you have enjoyed good health all your life, attributing to chance what has been secured and can only be maintained by science, effort, and the wise use of money. In the Churchillian triad of blood, sweat, and tears, you seem to haggle over expending too much sweat (or money) and forget the immense spiritual and vital economy of being spared the tears and the blood. It is time for modern man to realize that medical care is already as important as food, housing, and clothing in the preservation as well as the enjoyment of life. City life obviously depends on water and food brought in from the country. But, far more significantly, city life depends on medical knowledge for the safeness of that food and drink and for the protection against epidemics that in the past have evacuated the cities in superstitious and bewildered panic.

Please do not conclude that I argue for medical protection and care as the *summum bonum* of existence. Man cannot live by bread alone, even when it is whole wheat and reinforced with minerals and all the known vitamins. There are greater ends in living than health. These ends can be attained by those who are not even in perfect health. The same is true of food, housing, and clothing—not particularly rewarding as ends in themselves, but, like health, of considerable importance as means to whatever ends you may deem worthy of living for. In claiming that health is as important as food, shelter, and clothing, I do not imply that it is more important, nor even that health is as important as truth, beauty, or love. But I like to imagine that at the end of a year's prosaic labors in a hookworm campaign in, say, South America, a public health officer encountered a seller of musical instruments who said, "*Senhor Doutor*, I thank you for your work, because I have sold this year more violins and guitars in this village than ever before, because now the people are well enough to sing." Though different races find each other's arts, philosophies, and religions not always acceptable, there is a notable amount of agreement everywhere that health wherewith to follow and practice them is good.

Quite as interesting as the advance in our control of disease, and perhaps as significant for the future, our interpretation of disease, and consequently our ways of reacting to it, have changed. In the past more than once they have changed, and usually in the direction of a less superstitious and more rational attitude. As the concept of disease has become more rational, it has involved, in one form or another, the recognition of how wise it is for the individual to be concerned with the health of others, as an aid to his own safety. Scientific knowledge of communicable disease demonstrated beyond any question the social aspects of individual illness, and the importance to one and all of a healthy common environment.

And now we are at the dawn of general, public, and widespread recognition that Great Medicine can deliver health more dependably, in a larger number of diseases, over a longer span of life, and to a larger number of people than it ever has been able to do before. But this cannot be without more money than used to be spent when we didn't know how to apply money to get health protection. Our first reaction to the increased cost of medical care could be summarized as being critical. To learn that the cost of medical care is increasing arouses feelings of resentment, petulance, doubt, studied indifference, skeptical challenge, cynical suspicion, genuine concern, bewildered alarm, and energetic curiosity. Several forces affect this reaction to the cost of medical care, some making the issue more urgent

How are medical education and care paid for?

and some masking the natural steps by which medical care has come to cost so much.

Of these forces let us name a few. The present inflation increases the per diem cost of hospital care and places the cost of medical education in the class of luxuries available only to a few even though its quality is now threatened with accelerating deterioration. The military needs of the euphemistically labeled "cold war" not only extend the period before the medical student can earn his expected living but diminish, meanwhile, the services of doctors and nurses to the civilian population and tend to raise the costs of adequate medical care. The available improvements and refinements of diagnosis and treatment involve elaborate and costly instruments and equipment as well as the special training and services of persons who know how to use them. The layman who complains of the cost of an electrocardiogram to decide whether or not the pain in his chest is due to coronary disease does not realize that fifty years ago, though coronary disease certainly existed, it had not even been described, much less recognized; nor was there any instrument such as the electrocardiograph. The old family physician could guess that something was wrong with the heart, but all the advantages of precise knowledge—and they are considerable—were lacking, so the treatment was as vague and variant as the knowledge that lay behind it. I am confident that given the facts, the layman would pay for today's medicine gladly if he knew that a sensible way lies at hand to do so. But at the present time there is an appalling lag of the laity, an appalling distance between the potentialities of Great Medicine and the actual application and use of those potentialities. If a sensible way lies open before us, what is it?

How are medical education and care paid for?

Prepayment on the basis of insurance is the way. If insurance is applicable against the losses of death, which is inevitable, by how much more is insurance applicable against the losses of avoidable disease? No evidence exists that life insurance as such has stopped people from dying. But there is incontrovertible proof that the application of medical science has eliminated the occurrence in various countries of a long array of diseases and dramatically reduced the incidence of others. The stark inevitability of death has made death easy to reckon with—at least on the insurance principle. Death is a single, visible, permanent, and undeniable reality. But illness seems less definite, less verifiable, more unpredictable, more variant—not absolute like death, but relative and often transitory and negligible. Death is absolute, unique, and certain; illness is relative, multiform, and seems fortuitous. Except in murder, war, capital punishment, and suicide, death requires no collaborators; sickness calls for, and from time immemorial has received, help from others, whether they be guided by superstitious terror, compassionate charity, or medical science. From such contrasts it is easy to see that disease presents to the human mind a far more complicated concept with which to reckon than does death. This, I suppose, is the reason why insurance against death has easily become a vast and exact business, while insurance against illness, like a creature struggling to emerge from its chrysalis, is caught in a strait jacket of tradition, ignorance, inadaptability, and fatalism. I am tormented to watch so slow an emergence, knowing what Great Medicine could do if it were only freed to move and grow. That is the purpose of this book: to help to free Great Medicine, if only in the minds of a small number of readers, to emerge from its chrysalis. No well-trained physician can contemplate the cribbed, cabined, and confined potentialities of medical science without making the choice between protest and cynicism, between action and apathy, as a way to adjust that vision to the wretched realities of today.

Nor is the struggling emergence of Great Medicine a mere spectacle to stare at. We have in these times far too many spectator sports, far too many bystanders who claim the word innocent—innocent bystanders—witnessing struggles, conveniently aloof. The doctors themselves, as well as the laymen, have some struggling to do. It seems to me the doctors should devote more energy to reducing the prevalent ignorance. We should spend more effort adapting ourselves to the certain needs, rather than the floundering demands, of human beings. And laymen should reexamine their conservative, traditional ways of thinking about disease and rid themselves of fatalism.

Fatalism? Yes, the modern form of fatalism that attributes good health to good luck and believes disease a matter of chance. Instead of courses in high school geometry given in the world today, I would like to see a course in the mathematics of probability. This I say in the hope of mending the present discrepancy between our ability to deal with certainties like death and our bewilderment in dealing with probabilities like disease or freedom from disease. We are so ill at ease with probabilities that in many a credo we insist that certain phenomena possess a certainty they do not have, when really we are talking merely of what are not certainties but only probabilities. Our own insecurity in life's varying probabilities provides the wry humor of Samuel Butler's observation that the art of living consists of being able to form adequate conclusions from inadequate evidence.

If you wish to reflect upon the reliability of common sense in matters of chance, I can digress for a moment with a simple question to which the common sense of most people proves a guide that is just picturesque in its unreliability. At a cocktail party for twenty persons, what do you think are the chances that two of the guests will prove to have the same birthday—not born in the same year but on the same day of the same month? Well, the chance is better than fifty-fifty; in fact, it is 52.05 percent. In the light of your incredulity on this point, you will forgive me, I hope, for suspecting that some very fuzzy thinking attends your assumptions regarding the probabilities of your falling ill (*absit omen!*) this year. Indeed, I would say *thy* assumptions regarding the probabilities of *thy* falling ill, for when the English language gave up the use of "thee" and "thou" and "thy," it became impossible for lecturers to speak exclusively to anyone but the Almighty.

But to return to the theme of unfettering Great Medicine so that it may meet human need. I mentioned getting rid of tradition. To Elton Mayo I am indebted for the realization that today we live in an adaptive culture, not a traditional one. What traditions have we to tell us the wise use of television, of jet planes, of atomic energy, of modern medical science? The advances of technology go beyond the experience gathered and distilled from the past. That modern technology transcends tradition is just another commonplace whose certainty is equaled only by our neglect of its implications. Our culture is not traditional, or, more precisely said, our present culture is not entirely traditional.

Indeed, much of the confusion and bewilderment today comes from the mixture and the conflict between the traditional elements of our culture and the adaptive measures we must devise and try in order to meet today's realities that are unprovided for by our traditions. Nor is the conflict made any more sensible by our divorcing Reason to marry Hate—turning our hatred of our own bewilderment into a hatred of other persons and groups.

Now loyalty to the same tradition and sharing the same values produce a sense of companionship, communion, solidarity, stability, and even a sense of being in the presence of Truth. All these feelings are so reassuring and pleasant as to become precious to the point of indispensability. As Francis Delaisi pointed out in 1927 in his remarkable book, *Les Contradictions du Monde moderne*,[1] mankind has risked life itself in defense of institutions considered to be essential to security and traditionally invested with the sense of companionship, communion, solidarity, and stability. So if we essay to reexamine any traditional aspects of the practice of medicine, as they may now bear upon the advent of some new basis for providing medical care, we can add decency to sagacity by realizing that such a reexamination could well proceed with the maximum of detachment, sympathy, and concern for the anxieties it may alert, as well as the errors it may contain.

Nonetheless, experience with other aspects of living suggests that the most serious as well as the most elusive difficulties are those masked by the odor of sanctity, and that some odd passengers get aboard and hide themselves on trains of the utmost respectability. If traditions, like people,

---

[1] Francis Delaisi, *Les Contradictions du Monde moderne* (Paris, Payot, 1927).

have the defects of their own qualities, perhaps we can discover their most elusive defects by deliberately reexamining their most unchallenged qualities.

One of the fine traditions of the practice of medicine, which may be giving shelter to something quite unsatisfactory, is the tradition of charity. Charity, like a loving mother, may override the rights of others in the protective solicitude, not to say the selflessly selfish ambition, she has for her own. Operating as charities, the hospitals have accepted or demanded, in the name of charity, the services of nurses, interns, and even patients in ways and to a degree that raise, at least retrospectively, questions as to who was giving what and in whose name. The time and care that nurses and interns have given hospital patients were required in the name of education and dispensed in the name of charity. Patients were called charity cases, but if they were used for teaching, it was not so often explained to them that this improved their care as that it was justified as a substitute for hospital fees. Doctors, for all that hospital positions enlarged their experience and enhanced their professional prestige, gave an enormous amount of time and effort in the name of charity. Even universities were expected to contribute to the care of the sick poor, which was charity though usually charged and considered as education. This somewhat elaborate set of interlocking masquerades needs to be understood if what used to be charity cases are now going to appear at hospitals with the cost of hospitalization, as they believe, already paid for by insurance premiums. Without charity zigzagging unchallenged in and out of the debit columns of hospital accounts, as it had in the past, and with nurses, interns, doctors, patients, and universities quietly observing the increasing rarity of charity patients, it will not be surprising if it will soon cost even more to run hospitals. And there will be further confusion and need for clear thinking, because even with its charity patients gone, a hospital will never be a purely business enterprise, to be judged exactly like a hotel keeper's or a merchant's or manufacturer's business. Neither in a store nor a factory nor a hotel is the purchaser uniformly in the same state of anxiety, uncertainty, dependence, and incapacity that afflicts the purchaser of hospital care. An essential element, albeit psychological, is dropping out of hospital accounting. Consequently, it seems to me that one of the noblest and most nearly unimpeachable traditions of medical care—the charity motive—will need dispassionate and realistic review simply because it was one of the immediate forerunners of prepayment plans that now in large measure obviate charity.

But prepayment plans will encounter their most dangerous and decisive tests in meeting the educational needs of the medical and paramedical professions. Now, a set of relationships, no matter how proficient it may be temporarily, deserves no confidence unless it is self-renewing. Organisms without any reproductive capacities are evidently sterile affairs, and all their functions are eclipsed by the certainty of their extinction. What serious claim can be sustained for a system of medical care that fails to produce persons who will carry it on in the future, or even for a system of medical care in which the doctors, the nurses, the public health officers, the dentists, the administrators, the technicians, nutritionists, special therapists—indeed, the health professions as a whole—will gradually deteriorate in point of the quantity and quality of service rendered to an increasingly needy population? Of the three characteristics of living tissue—adaptation, growth, and reproduction—the last, reproduction, provides the most searching question to be asked if we want to test for vitality and continuity. Keepers of zoos begin to feel at ease when their more exotic animals succeed in producing their own kind in captivity. Since medical education replenishes the professions that provide medical care, and since medical care is changing in important ways, we must be on guard to make sure that none of the new factors or practices of medical care threatens the continuity of medical education.

I would draw your particular attention to the following statement: *The cost of medical education is a part of the cost of medical care.* This is one of those axiomatic truths whose implications and corollaries run far beyond those seen at first glance. Let us then examine more closely the meaning of the statement.

Like any kind of education, medical education involves outlays of time, effort, and money, and it takes time to repay the investor, whether it is the pupil, the teacher, the parent, or society at large which is considered the investor in medical education. In short, education calls for time, and in order to understand education one must have a framework of time, a sense of its passage, and, above all, an awareness of the future. Medical care in the future depends on medical education in the present. Today's teaching controls tomorrow's practice. With few qualifications, one can say that the medical care of today derives from the medical education of previous decades. It is a peculiar kind of dependent, sequential relationship. We could close every medical school and hospital for a year or, perhaps, for five years without entirely stopping medical care for any corresponding one- or five-year period in the future. The neighboring generations of doctors would in neighborly fashion cover the gap. But a stoppage or a deterioration of education over a longer period would prove of unimaginable and all but irremediable harm. It proves nothing to learn that in 1857 the endowment of Randolph-Macon College was but a few thousand dollars less than that of Harvard, but it starts us to thinking on the spreading losses of the war between the States. Nor do we have to go so far back to find examples of the effects of war in wrecking education and thus producing later the characteristic patterns of hopelessness, apathy, and cynicism.

The cost of medical education can be regarded on still other grounds as part of the cost of medical care, and this without any involvement of the future whatever. Medical education actually is part of medical care wherever medical education is going on. Hospital trustees are beginning to recognize the truth of what was only regarded as an educational hypothesis thirty years ago, namely, that affiliation with a medical school means the opportunity for a hospital to give better service than is otherwise possible. Indeed, such affiliation with medical education has recently provided some hospitals in Britain with a privileged status, exempted their endowments from absorption by the government, and proved that medical education is a remarkably vital element in medical care; indeed, teaching activities offer a hospital the best guarantee of its continuity. The educational devices we call internships and residencies, after struggles of varying length and intensity on the part of their sponsors, who were interested in education, have long since become indispensable in the task of providing medical care. At present the storm center of criticism and opposition is the education of nurses. One would have expected more prompt recognition of the fact that the education of nurses is a part of the cost of medical care, if only because nursing care in many a hospital has long been made possible by the simple but somewhat disingenuous device of setting up a school of nursing and stringing out the course so that enough work was gotten out of pupil nurses to run the hospital, as well as pay for the niggardly salaries of teachers and the mediocre teaching facilities offered them in the name of education.

The bald fact is that the cost of first-rate medical care in many of the teaching hospitals of the United States is being paid by universities. An element of fairness would be introduced if the universities were paid for such services instead of paying so much for the opportunity to give them. One of the immense advantages that could accrue from applying prepayment insurance to defray the cost of medical care is the relief it would bring to university budgets from the heavy burden of caring for the improvident sick. If caring for the improvident sick be advanced as a legitimate charge on higher education, then I can only expect the more intelligent among the highly educated eventually to repudiate such claims. It really is high time to get the costs of medical care clarified, properly recorded, and accepted for what they actually are.

But it will be a grim day for the future of medical care when prepayment plans forget that the cost of education is a part of the cost of care. No doubt, medical care will become more expensive. As a friend of mine observed ruefully, "My children never cost me much until they became independent." In somewhat the same way I expect that when the eleemosynary confusion is removed from medical care, and when those involved in it begin to ask for remuneration, as I think they will as the charity argument declines, we shall find that being our own keepers costs somewhat more than the amiable but somewhat confused business of being our brother's keeper. Indeed, there will be some surprises in store for us when we become our brother's bookkeeper. Perhaps the crowning surprise of all will be to find that being our brother's keeper and bookkeeper—that is, looking after each other and knowing exactly what this costs—pays, and pays increasingly. For the increase in health that the sensible application of Great Medicine offers would entrain a surprising increase in our total earning power and wealth. From this increased wealth it would be easier to maintain prepayment insurance policies. And with better medical care we should witness a decreasing incidence of disease among dependent children and among ourselves throughout the wage-earning period.

Of the declining years I am less certain. If we are prolonging the years of mere existence, we run the risk of trading mortality for morbidity, of lasting longer, yes, but with more infirmity to care for. Sometimes, amid campaigns against so many diseases we don't want to die of, I think, somewhat flippantly, that we might sensibly focus our attention on deciding which among several mortal diseases we do like, which exits we prefer; and, in dignified acceptance of the inevitable, we might depart after perhaps less stampeding and general confusion.

But let us return to the theme of prepayment. What is its present status? It is growing. Indeed, it is already widely spread and growing fast, so fast as to remind me of a story that has long been my solace when the buzz of argument about prepayment is ringing in my ears. The story is of a man who, before the days of the tunnels and bridges to the Jersey side of the Hudson, found himself desperately late to catch the last ferry boat at night. As he rushed down the slip, he saw there was already eight feet of open water between the slip and the boat. He threw his suitcase on board, called to the crowd to stand back, took a run and a jump, and landed in a heap on the ferry boat. And as he stood up, a sailor tapped him on the shoulder, saying, "Say, what's the matter with you? Didn't you know this boat was coming in?"

It is not whether prepayment is coming in or not that has been worrying me. I want it to come in without smashing the boat or the pier—without injuring the effectiveness of the health professions or harming the consumers and beneficiaries of medical care. As between ship and pier, the pier seems to me to offer the sturdier planks and the more nearly final resistance. No profession can afford to ignore, or try to crush, the opinions and sentiments of its clients. They won't crush! I would therefore think it sensible to make a few remarks on the consumers of medical care.

The attitude of individuals toward prepayment for medical care is usually inarticulate, or articulate only through various types of associations to which they belong. To these associations I will refer in a moment. The doctor-patient relationship in times of anxiety is so intimate, and in times of evident peril so tense, that no one can overlook the psychological importance of the patient's freedom to choose his own doctor. Indeed, whenever the charge can be laid against any form of the practice of medicine that it precludes or obstructs the free choice of doctor, the accuser scores a point. But it is a point that would carry more weight with me if laymen showed more intelligence in the exercise of this freedom and if in many a small town or farm area there were more than one doctor to choose from. I would also be more impressed on this point if laymen, prepared to pay for their own care, never went long distances to hospitals and clinics to put themselves in the care of an institution without knowing a single member of its staff, and if I hadn't seen such excellent and conscientious care given by doctors who were not chosen by their patients. I do not deny, however, that free choice of doctor is important and desirable; what I deny is that it is in practice or in theory indispensable. But I will admit that as a specious argument against group practice, teaching hospitals, and the theory of prepayment for medical care, it has a distressingly meretricious appeal. But perhaps it is wasted emotion to be anxious about the possible abuse of the argument of freedom of choice of doctor, as it has borne on the advancement of schemes depending on prepayment. Certainly the growth of Blue Cross and Blue Shield, and of insurance companies in the same field, suggests that no amount of raising the question of the free choice of doctor is likely to stop the progress of health insurance.

The chief concern that I feel about the individual and his attitude toward prepayment centers around his probable ignorance of what a great protection it is to him to be used for teaching. On that point we must all focus our imaginations, our solicitude, and our educational endeavors. Since teaching on private patients has been done successfully for years at the Billings Hospital of the University of Chicago, and has been done in steadily increasing measure in most of our teaching hospitals, there is no cause for concern except on two points: that patients and their doctors will prefer the nonteaching hospitals and that the trustees of such non-teaching hospitals will refrain from medical school affiliation, preferring a high bed occupancy to the opportunity to give better care. The private practitioner without a teaching appointment has usually been willing to turn over to a teaching hospital a patient he could not afford to treat gratis. By so much as the patients formerly of this category provide themselves with health insurance, the non-teaching hospitals will increase their bed occupancy. We shall have busier doctors, but there is a danger that the teaching of the next generation of doctors will suffer. Where can the medical schools turn to obtain for their students adequate experience with an appropriate number of patients?

Through making affiliations with medical schools the Veterans Administration, thanks to the admirable character and distinguished abilities of General Paul R. Hawley, M.D., and Dr. Elliot C. Cutler and the support of General Omar N. Bradley, has given an example of improving medical care by introducing teaching into the work of the V.A. hospitals. By so much as these accomplishments and arrangements are slighted or skimped in the future, it is the patients who will suffer promptly as well as eventually, verifiably though less clearly. Continuing vigilance will be required to maintain the level set by General Hawley. In return for what they give the V.A. patients, the medical schools can increase their clinical resources.

Furthermore, as long as the claims of the veterans for care for non-service-connected disabilities provide an incalculable uncertainty to reckon with, we can be sure of only two facts: (1) that the present number of veterans—roughly 22,000,000, and in the spring of 1953 growing at the rate of about 45,000 a month—is each year approaching the years of increased infirmity and decreased earning power and (2) that free medical care for veterans provides on a seriously large scale the most inviting alternative to prepayment plans for a considerable portion of the adult population. Perhaps one could add that if the demand for medical care from the Veterans Administration does not increase over the next four decades, the only reason will have been the effective competition of prepayment plans. Of course, a tragic deterioration in the care given could widely discredit the Veterans Administration, but that cannot occur unknown to the medical school representatives, or go unprotested if they retain their integrity.

As between compulsory prepayment for medical care and voluntary prepayment plans, I prefer the voluntary type. Granted that complete and prompt coverage of the entire population could be obtained only by a uniform, nationwide, compulsory system, I still would prefer prepayment to be on a voluntary basis. Why? Because compulsory prepayment plans would have to be more uniform, less varied, and more centrally controlled than the voluntary type.

Now, I happen to be convinced that variety is much more than the spice of life: variety comes very near to being the most reliable guarantee of survival that we possess. Life is forever trying new combinations, different arrangements, various experiments. I don't think we know enough about the complicated forces and facts of health insurance to risk much on any one uniform or centrally administered plan. Among all imaginable kinds of freedom, the freedom to vary, to differ, to try, seems to me the most precious. We should be mad to expect that numerous and varied prepayment plans for medical care would offer little and prove nothing of value as our experience with their virtues and defects increases.

Furthermore, a number of variant, independent prepayment plans would require more discussion, cooperation, and understanding than a general compulsory scheme. Also, conditions in different parts of the country would distort any one scheme into a strange congeries of actual effects and thus defeat the very uniformity we supposed we were obtaining.

No serious evidence can be presented that in their present numbers the medical and paramedical personnel in this country could meet the requirements of a uniform, obligatory health insurance plan. Such a plan would be too big to deal with. We shall have to experiment, beginning where beginnings are possible, finding our way, and insisting on the absolutely fundamental essentiality of variety.

The two greatest factors in favor of prepayment for medical care are now coming into view with power and impatience. The labor unions, the C.I.O., and the A.F. of L., see medical care and health benefits as a form of recompense whose cost they would like to see deducted from pay checks and, thus, collected as prepayment. Similarly, the three major organizations of farmers are naturally concerned with the quality of medical care available to rural populations. Furthermore, they are not among the most credulous when told that it is already excellent. By so much as prepayment plans can be shown to meet rural needs, the farmers' organizations will support such plans. And they will do so with scant regard for the more traditional forms of medical care that can hardly be said to give them a present glow of satisfaction.

Now, with some of the circumstances, implications, advantages, and characteristics of prepayment in mind as a means for paying for medical care, let us ask for *l'addition, s'il vous plaît, die Rechnung, bitte*, and pick up the check.

Having in mind a prepayment that would eventually carry medical education adequately for the paramedical professions as well as for doctors, that also would provide for a steadily increasing population, that would cover obsolescence as well as maintenance of our hospitals, and that would give broad and simplified coverage for everything (including eventually mental disease and tuberculosis) and still leave some funds for research, let me set up a figure of $100 a year per capita as the premium for health insurance. That is a little less than $2.00 a week, or $8.33 a month. That seems a figure obviously beyond the range of a vast majority of the population. For a family of five on an annual income of $3,000, the sum of $500 would seem at present an impossibly large fraction of their total income to devote to health insurance. But our 156 million citizens spend $4,300,000,000 on cigarettes; that means an annual average of $27.50 per capita—and not everybody smokes. Comparing that $27.50 for cigarettes with the $26.16 I pay for hospital insurance brings into sharp relief the one point I want to insist on: we do not yet regard prepayment plans at anywhere near their real value.

To argue that $100 a year per capita is a reasonable premium for health insurance would make no sense at all if it were a figure to be applied to compulsory prepayment for everyone. But one of the advantages of voluntary prepayment plans is that they offer variety and adaptability to different groups. The time has come for groups of laymen who can afford $8.33 a month per capita for health insurance to find out what extraordinary values they could get for such a relatively trivial outlay. At present we expect medical care to thrive in spite of our reluctance. It won't, because it can't.

98   *How are medical education and care paid for?*

I do not wish to exhaust your patience or abuse your attention with a long exposition on medical economics and of intricate estimates. Indeed, I want to use this opportunity in quite a different way. I want to point out that in the light of what medicine has done and can do for us, our reluctance to pay more—much more—for medical care and protection is simply fantastic. My point, in briefest form, is that the table of life that traditionally has rested on the tripod of food, clothing, and shelter can now rest more securely and more reasonably on four legs—food, clothing, shelter, and medical care. The last and newest leg cannot sensibly be much shorter or weaker than the others. Keeping well and alive has become, without our realizing it, part of one's living expenses. We shall solve nothing by insisting that if we must spend $2.00 a day or more on food we cannot afford 28 cents a day for medical care. We shall get to no pleasant destination by improvidence or by regarding medical protection as an avoidable luxury.

What boarding house will keep you above starvation for $2.00 a week? But that amount may protect you from a life of dependency and invalidism if it secures for you hospital care at the crucial moment. And monthly room rents begin, for the majority, at figures above $8.33 a month —where per capita health insurance leaves off.

Frankly, I think that some of our health insurance plans are too timid. They have the timidity of the early manufacturers of iceboxes, who spent all their energies trying to make iceboxes cheaper, only to learn that what the housewives wanted was better iceboxes that were good and not cheaper iceboxes that were bad. I think the time has come for a $100 per capita prepayment project to find out how much it can do, rather than a $26.16 per capita plan to be troubled and handicapped by how little it can offer.

In short, I cannot believe that in this country at the present time there is not a very large number of persons who could afford 28 cents a day for a kind of medical care far superior to anything we have yet had in prepayment plans. Twenty-eight cents a day provides $102.20 a year. With such a revenue per capita, our prepayment organizations could offer, as time goes on, an increasing measure of protection and an example that would become more and more attractive to a larger and larger number of subscribers.

In essence, my theme is this: the layman does not realize that modern medicine could bring him immense advantages if only he would consider health in a sensible perspective relative to the other expenses of keeping alive. A practical way lies open now to take advantage of what Great Medicine could do for us. Voluntary prepayment is the path, and each one of us could be a pathfinder and a contributor to a great new development.

5. The natural history of the doctor

IN many a discussion of social change, of institutional reform or adjustment, of the effect of new forces and new alignments on existing professions, I frequently miss any reference to a most important item, namely, the kind of people that are involved. Such terms as "Great Medicine" and "disease" are both abstract and collective; the "medical and paramedical professions" represents a collective phrase with a very considerable measure of inclusiveness and scope. A teacher I had in college, Professor Edwin B. Holt, once pointed out to me a fact of considerable bearing when one is dealing with abstract and collective nouns. "A word," he said, "that has many connotations can denote nothing; conversely, a word that denotes but one thing has no connotations." The word water, for example, has numerous connotations—"weak as water," "As the hart panteth after the water books," "as wet as water," etc.—but H_2O denotes but one thing and so has no connotations.

Now, it seems to me that part of the task of the poet or the essayist is to use the connotative words that exactly convey his feeling, whereas a part of the task of the scientist is to employ denotative words with comparable logical skill and verifiable precision. In something approximating an essay on the place of the art and science of medicine today, I feel restless to have employed abstract and collective terms

The natural history of the doctor

so often and in apparent disregard of the kind of people, or, better, the kinds of people, that doctors are. For a word such as "medicine" has many connotations, from which different hearers will choose different meanings. And since, as Oscar Wilde remarked, "All criticism is a form of autobiography," I venture to think that one useful step in understanding where medicine belongs today might well take the form of an essay on "The Natural History of the Doctor." For the doctor's criticisms and his attitudes derive in considerable measure from his personal experiences, so if there be anything generic or even somewhat uniform in the background and experience of doctors, then by studying the doctor's professional experiences we should have further understanding of their professional attitudes and behavior.

I propose to present, first, the paradigm or at least some of the characteristic features of the life story of the young doctor in the United States today and then offer some comment on what I have noted as the usual experiences in the natural history of young doctors of today elsewhere in the world. I shall try to distinguish between what I know are my personal opinions and, on the other hand, statements generally reported or agreed upon as accepted facts.

Beginning with the families in America that provide recruits to the medical profession, one can safely say that they are usually middle class and, if one uses Lloyd Warner's system of class notation, upper middle class. Perhaps one could say that only rarely does a boy who is certain to inherit a large fortune choose to go into medicine. At the other end of the income spectrum, the number of boys eager to be doctors but whose parents could not afford to carry them through a long and expensive form of education is far larger than we realize. We should have a slightly clearer idea of the great potentialities of this second group if a larger number of our colleges had scholarships like the Cope Scholarships at Haverford, which provide each year funds for three years of professional schooling, not at Haverford, but elsewhere, to one senior graduating from Haverford. Such college-leaving scholarships aid the college to attract earnest students because of the chance they offer students of going further. So clearly desirable an award stimulates the students while in college. Such scholarships aid the professional schools because the college committee of award knows the candidates' performance intimately, broadly, and over four years and, furthermore, wants to pick a good representative of the college. The winner of the award is likely to feel an added sense of responsibility as the chosen representative of his college. The experience at Haverford with this type of scholarship has confirmed all these theoretical assumptions. If only for the benefit the medical schools would gain by competing with other graduate schools, I would like to see most colleges in this country able to give one or more college-leaving scholarships. But let us remember that a profession we might like to see free from any preoccupation with money finds its very recruitment shadowed, and the earlier years of its members preoccupied, with financial risks and economic success.

The essential point is that, almost uniformly, boys choosing a medical career know that they will have to earn their living from it. They also know that the preliminary cost in time, effort, and money before they can be self-supporting will be heavier than it would be for any other professional career. At one of our large medical schools on the eastern seaboard, the class graduated in 1953 reported that 60 percent of its members were married and that the average annual cost of living and going to medical school was $3,640 for a married couple and $2,260 for a single student. The wives of most of the married students were gainfully employed and making an essential contribution to their husband's chance at a professional career—not vaguely helpmeets but very definitely help-meet-expenses. Such enterprise and fortitude result quite naturally in the resolve as well as the necessity of looking for a professional income later that will enable them to justify the outlay and to repay such loans as they may have obtained. The proportion of medical students who have received so-called G.I. benefits after military service now begins to fall off rapidly in our medical schools, and I can't help expressing regret and foreboding that we shall see an increasing limitation, almost entirely for economic reasons, of admirable recruits to the medical profession. Aptitude and longing to enter this career are so widespread that I can but regret the frustration.

Obviously, the decision to go to medical school can now but rarely be impulsive, hasty, or unreflecting. Indeed, Frank Boyden of Deerfield Academy told me once that medicine stands out among all careers as being the one that schoolboys select early and with a manifest clarity of preference. I have posed to a good many doctors the question, "How old were you when you decided that you wanted to be a doctor?" and though there have been plenty of exceptions, the majority has confirmed the impression that the decision is often made early. If this be true, there are probably some interesting aspects of the subject of motivation in the choice of a medical career.

It is my personal impression that boys choose medicine for one or more of three reasons and occasionally go to medical school because of a fourth. The first reason is that they sense the nature of the doctor's relationship with people and like it. They sense the intimacy of that relationship and the mystery of it, the good that doctors do, and the respect and affection in which doctors often seem to be held. The second motive is perhaps not precisely a motive but rather a susceptibility or field of interest; it shows in the boy who loves animals, keeps pets, and prefers rambling in the countryside, or a visit to the zoo, to any other use of his time. He is at heart a biologist. He stands transfixed by the contemplation of living things, and, as his mind becomes more mature, he is fascinated by the phenomena and the mysteries of human life. The third motive relates to the power and composure, the prestige, and sometimes the evident ease and wealth of the doctor. Such authority any child can feel without putting it in so many words. Like the primary colors, which are rarely seen in nature unmixed, these motives, combined in one or another individual proportion, seem to me to compose the primary reasons for the choice of a medical career. There is, of course, a fourth reason, but it can hardly claim consideration as a motive. Some boys are so harried by their parents to become doctors that they go to medical school in default of any other tastes or interests strong enough to withstand parental pressures. When you see such students—and such doctors—you can be sorry for them, but you can regret even more that they have taken a place desired by others who would have brought a deeper interest and a happier devotion to the practice of medicine. I would be sorrier for those who go into medicine against their own will had I not seen examples of the deftness they can use in avenging themselves. One young man I knew, who was forced into studying medicine when he preferred music, completed medical school and then became organist of the Church of Christ, Scientist.

Most observers who know secondary schools on both sides of the Atlantic would agree, I think, that the quality of our secondary school education in terms of preparation for college, to be followed by professional schools, leaves a good deal to be desired. It seems wasteful of time, lacking in thoroughness, and somewhat confused in objective. One understands some of the reasons for this on learning that in the seventy-year interval between 1870 and 1940 the general population in the United States increased only threefold, the college enrollment, thirtyfold, while the secondary school enrollment increased ninetyfold. So rapid an expansion enhances the likelihood of confusion of objectives and dilution of standards.

Even if a boy decides on medicine before entering college, it is not until he enters college that he begins to see the early but concrete implications of that decision. His college courses must include those required or advised for the premedical student. The courses required in chemistry, physics, and biology do not, generally speaking, make, in and of themselves, any unreasonable demand. But the student is likely to misinterpret the statement that a defined amount of study in these subjects is required for entrance. Unfortunately, he may infer that the more of just these three subjects he takes the larger will be his chance of being admitted to medical school. As a result he narrows his horizons, intensifies his efforts in physics, chemistry, and biology and limits the amount of his general cultural baggage during precisely the three or four years that offer the last chance of a liberal education. Sometimes he takes an excessive proportion of courses in physics, chemistry, and biology, out of a perfectly honest but sometimes unreflecting preference for just those subjects. Or, as a curiously sophomoric compromise, he loads the first two or three college years with physics, chemistry, and biology, under the naïve assumption that he can pick up the cultural subjects in senior year. The result is that such fields as English (including the ability to express himself in something approximating that language), mathematics, history, government, the fine arts, philosophy, modern languages, psychology, and sociology he views hurriedly and superficially, if at all. He fails to realize that cultivation in these fields is hardly a brisk "spit and polish" job, and hurried maturity is a denial in terms.

The effect of the present deferment from military service of premedical students while they are in college sharply intensifies the competitive side of their college work. It is, as the students say, "a rat race, with Uncle Sam breathing down your neck every time you walk into an examination room." For if you don't get accepted by a medical school, you are subject to draft—and the applicants for admission to medical schools have recently outnumbered those admitted, by about twenty-seven to ten. The tensions of this competition are bad enough, but they cause less permanent loss to the contestants than does the deliberate restriction of the students' horizons. That restriction calls for remedy.

A. N. Whitehead once remarked that he knew of no professional degree that opens to its holder the opportunity to exercise as wide a range of talents and tastes as that afforded by the M.D. degree. If we cannot deny the truth of that opinion, it would certainly be natural to wonder whether the present stipulations as to chemistry, physics, and biology could not profit from being better understood, together with the value of a broader general education than they offer. The plan of allowing 5 percent of the entering class to be admitted to medical school without presenting exactly the educational experience required of the remaining 95 percent has much in its favor. As an example, it has produced an electrifying effect on the admissions committee in raising such questions as what kinds of individual excellences are more interesting for a medical school to encourage than just maintaining a uniformity of training in the entering class.

Admission to medical schools in the United States is commonly based on marks obtained in college courses, certain aptitude tests, and a personal interview with one or more members of the medical school's admissions committeee. In point of the purely scholastic records, I know of medical schools that apply a specific system of discounts on the marks given by each college. They have derived these discounts from experience with the graduates of the different colleges. This they do because a performance that might receive an A-minus in a college with poor standards would obtain only C-plus in another. Because any and all refined quantification of what happens in higher education seems to me specious, if not, indeed, spurious, I would prefer the less precise guarantee of intellectual ability implied by the requirement that the medical school applicant stand in the upper half, third, or quarter of his college class (the smaller the class the larger the fraction).

The psychological tests offer, perhaps, an occasional warning regarding an individual applicant, but in the main they seem to me to be only broadly corroborative. In some instances it may sensibly be said that it is the tests that are still being tested rather than the candidates. Nonetheless, the selection of medical students, especially when those applying considerably outnumber those admitted, remains an unresolved problem of the greatest importance to the future of the profession.

If the ability to select capable doctors from among candidates for entrance to medical schools at all resembles the task of picking capable teachers from among candidates for instructorships, then I commend to your attention the record of President Cary Thomas of Bryn Mawr. She selected as instructors for their first teaching posts Jacques Loeb, the biologist; Thomas H. Morgan, the geneticist; E. B. Wilson, the cytologist; Elmer P. Kohler, the chemist; Franklin Giddings in sociology; and Woodrow Wilson in history and government. The performances of Hyde at Bowdoin, Eliot at Harvard, Harper at Chicago, and Gilman at Hopkins in picking future academic stars further prompts one to wonder whether the capacity to judge emergent ability and its probability of future high performance is not a human ability we should study as actively as we experiment with psychological tests. I would, for example, suggest that every teacher in the first two years' courses in a medical school be asked to give each of his students two marks: one for performance in the course and the other to represent the teacher's estimate of the student's probable subsequent performance as a student, intern, and resident. After a sufficient number of such marks had been correlated with actual experience, it would be easy to find among the teachers any exceptionally good judge of young men; and he should be put on the admissions committee, where his talent would be of irreplaceable value.

The personal interview suggests an aspect of medical student selection which has long interested me, and which claims no less attention as the demands increase in the practice of medicine for doctors possessed of what is called a social sense. The need for public-spirited doctors increases as the social significance of health grows. But as medical training lengthens and becomes more costly, the temptation to make money and commercialize the profession increases, too, and perhaps all the more so if the restraint imposed by charity work decreases as prepayment plans diminish the number of charity patients.

My suggestion is simple: it is that medical school admissions committees pay more attention to the character, records, and attitudes of the parents of applicants for admission. The suggestion is simple, but the reasons for the suggestion are not. They are, I should declare at the outset, quite personal, and though I have a few friends who hold much the same views, I have never seen such views put explicitly on record.

Just as there are some men who seek and obtain their greatest satisfactions in competition with others, so there are persons whose greatest satisfactions come not from competition but from the affectionate respect they can gain from others. Not only do such types exist, but they recur in family histories in a way that suggests that such predilections are familial, or possibly that they are hereditary. I used to think such noncompetitive individuals a little bit superior morally to the merely competitive type, but I have long since come to regard the socially minded as though they labored under a hereditary taint—they can't help themselves. They are, if you choose, selfish in their demand for the rewards of unselfishness. They crave gratitude and affection as hungrily as other men want to be envied or competitively successful. The socially minded help, it is true, to keep society together, but they usually forget that the more competitive type of man finds equal, if not more, exhilaration when he can regard his fellows as competitors or even enemies to be conquered. The ideals, the philosophies, the credos, and the heroes each type follows are actually the ones his innate tastes prompt him to select as further prods in the direction he already has chosen. If I hold, and I do, that the organization of the practice of medicine would benefit now from a little less of competitive commercialism and a little more sense for the public welfare, then that, too, is probably evidence of my tastes influencing my judgment. What do you hold?

We can move to somewhat less self-conscious ground if I call your attention to the remarkable frequency with which three professions have enriched their own and each other's ranks by breeding socially minded individuals—the teachers, the ministers, and the doctors. The German professorial families and the record in public service of the sons of the vicarage and the manse in Britain lend some support to my supposition that if social-mindedness be not influenced by heredity, it is at least strongly encouraged by the ideals and values in the families of teachers, ministers, and doctors. Is this an aristocratic or an undemocratic view? If so, that implies we think these poor folk, who are ridden with contributing to the comfort and gladness of mankind, are a superior cut, or that they wish to dominate. They don't; they want to serve. Are they aristocratic? That may be, but it is no part of my theory.

In application, the theory would simply come to this: If the medical profession seems to need a little larger mixture of persons who actually enjoy working for others, those charged with recruiting its ranks should give larger attention to candidates coming from homes where contributions to the public welfare have been the example set as well as where interest in the public welfare has been accorded attention, praise, admiration, and rewards. At present the admissions committees seem to me to give considerable weight to the candidate's mental abilities. Circumstances at present also favor the candidate whose purse matches his mind. But the general public complains of the scarcity of doctors controlled by compassion and public spirit, qualities nearer the heart than the mind or the purse.

The four years in medical school that used to cover most of a good medical education now make up only four-sevenths of it, and sometimes less than a half. The medical school introduces the student to an enormous range of facts and fields and skills and, under pressure from the licensing boards, essays to give a guarantee of competence to practice medicine at the end of the fourth year. Actually, the fourth year is about the time when the student is deciding what particular competence he will set out to acquire in the following one to five years. The four-year myth dies hard, but it is at least more nearly moribund than ever before, now that the armed forces prefer to wait till at least a fifth year has been completed in an internship, or even a sixth or seventh year in a residency. Thus the medical student who entered college at 17 leaves medical school at 24 or 25, but he is not yet experienced enough to take his full load of responsibilities as a doctor. For, to repeat what needs to be remembered, the Greeks grimly observed that there are only two kinds of men who can kill their fellows in peacetime with impunity: doctors and judges. It were well if the laity could see in that observation an argument for better medical schools. As the juries have taken over the judge's responsibility, so in some measure group practice helps to protect the individual doctor from making mistakes. But the stern responsibility of the individual doctor remains.

It is of more than passing interest that when the usual medical course was four years long, Abraham Flexner attacked the dominance of practitioners in the second half of that four-year course. He preferred full-time teachers. Now that the course is seven or eight years in actual practice, the influence of practitioners, through the requirements of specialty boards, has in considerable measure returned. The specialty boards set themselves up rather more as taskmasters than as teachers. If certification of specialists by the specialty boards claims praise for raising the general performance level of specialists in this country, that praise is deserved. But, if it claims credit as the ideal way to advance knowledge and competence in special fields, more trust could well be put in the medical schools for that task, if only they were decently supported to do it.

This is not the place for an extended discussion of the curriculum and the teaching methods and similar problems of medical education. But I would point out again that since there is too much factual knowledge and practical skill to impart in so short a period of time as four years, the part of wisdom seems to me to lie in training the student's capacities rather than stuffing his memory. What capacities? The capacity to observe, to reason, to compare his observations and reasoning with those of others, and the capacity to put himself in his patient's place—compassion. With such abilities trained, sharpened, and refined, the graduate of a medical school would find in his fifth, or intern year, and later as assistant resident and resident, the opportunities to use and refine those capacities to the immediate and the infinite advantage of his patients and himself.

But the really crucial period for the medical student comes at the very end of his preparatory experience. What decides the rest of his professional life is what he does after the internship or the residency is over. He then decides whether to stay in teaching and research or to leave it. He then considers offers from group clinics or older doctors who want a competent assistant. He then decides for or against permanent government service. At this point he has the offer or the desire to go to a community that needs a doctor. In short, at this point the die is cast. And I would add that I know of no money more effectively invested for the advantage of great Medicine than funds made available to medical schools to pay adequate salaries to hold the best qualified young men, at this stage, to careers in research and teaching. I could not possibly exaggerate the value of such assistance at this time.

This all-too-brief review of the natural history of the doctor in America today can be perhaps elaborated or given a setting by some remarks on the life history of a medical student in some other countries. Travel develops one's perception of the similarities and the uniformities as well as the differences and the exceptions and the peculiarities of different cultures.

To a degree that we do not realize, the years of secondary education in any country supply some unexpectedly significant elements in professional education. Of course, one cannot distinguish clearly the effects of home training and family tradition from the effects of the secondary school in preparing students for the higher ranges of professional responsibility, whether in practice, teaching, or research. It would be worse than invidious to name areas or countries to illustrate the opinions I am about to express, but on this score the large number of countries and areas from which the illustrations are drawn will serve to obviate that difficulty.

I believe it was Samuel Butler who said that one of the arts of living consists in the ability to come to adequate conclusions from inadequate evidence. In any event, much of our practical living involves action on the basis of assumptions of varying degrees of probability. We often forget, only to recall at leisure later, that the most improbable events are not impossible. They are only extremely improbable. In just this sense, I would think it highly improbable that medical students can wisely be expected to acquire for the first time at so late a stage in their preparation, basic intellectual honesty, industrious habits, dependable morality, or freedom from the shackles of tradition and authoritarianism if in neither home nor secondary school they have met examples of or training in honesty, responsibility, hard work, and freedom of mind and spirit. I do not think we often stop to realize how much of these qualities we assume to be present in medical students, nor how much we rely, unconsciously, on these qualities that are essential to the effectiveness of our institutions of higher learning.

I can think of countries where the authoritarian and traditional elements of the surrounding culture are so powerful that it appears to be excessively difficult for their young people either to entertain or assert any idea or observation that runs counter to the traditional beliefs or the current authorities. It is difficult enough for us; for them it is extremely improbable. It is not impossible, but can we expect a graduate student coming from such an environment, when exposed for a year or two to an atmosphere in which he is expected to show originality of mind and independence of spirit, to show promptly just what he has never before acquired or even encountered? I have known traveling fellows who were dumbfounded to be told by a professor that he expected them to express disagreement with him, provided they could give their evidence for holding a contrary opinion. I recall a medical scientist of the greatest distinction who told me that during his graduate fellowship year at one of the great English universities he encountered for the first time the idea that in scientific work one should be really honest in reporting the results of his experiments. Before that time he had always been told and had quite naturally assumed that the point was to get his observations and theories accepted by others, and published. As a less serious example of naïveté, I recall a student nurse from the upper classes of her country who, having dropped her handkerchief on the floor, stood waiting for a menial to come along to pick it up for her. I recall a country where even a well-supervised reading room for students offered too great a temptation to the students to steal textbooks, thus frustrating the hopes of the teachers to offer the students the chance to use a library widely. In short, I am inclined to believe that some of the less talked about essentials of medical education and reliable research are laid down not in medical schools but well before then. If this be a fact, then the expectedly effective transfer of the methods of medical education and research from one country to another may call for reflection and for measures that have not had the attention they deserve.

Discarding for the moment any efforts at a measure of

precision, which would only mislead us, we may say that during the first decade of life we learn to live in the world about us, that during much of the second decade we learn to live with our contemporaries as well as our elders, and that somewhere around the end of the second decade begins the task of learning to express ourselves in a medium of the culture in which we find ourselves, and to formulate our ideas of success and failure, of satisfaction, of the good life. All these periods and activities overlap each other. I mention them only to suggest that one of the unrecognized activities of the premedical and medical years is selecting and fixing, and more closely than ever before defining, the pattern of what we want to be and do, of what will satisfy us— in short, what we are learning to believe is the good life. For just that reason it will always be valuable for medical students to see and especially to know examples, and exemplars, of what a good doctor is. The students need ideals, but they need still more deeply to see that ideals can be incarnated and realized in a living man, because their immediate and their continuing task is to become what they want to be. Fortunate, indeed, is the medical school that possesses an example or two worth following, and if by chance it possesses a first-class exemplar like Francis W. Peabody, then the effect is almost miraculous and his influence for good all but legendary.

Though the maturity of the student determines in considerable measure how he will go through his experiences and what he will distill and retain from them, he encounters, in going into medical school, much the same generic experiences in any and every country. If for years he has looked forward to entering the medical school, he experiences on entrance a sense of satisfaction that swiftly turns to something like incredulous awe as he realizes the importance as well as the intricacy of the issues he must learn not only to face, but to take direction over. No more stark or eloquent reminder of such issues could be imagined than the dissection of a human body. Nor can it be denied that such an experience raises for many a student that whole congeries of questions and uncertainties we call the problem of death. I doubt if it is fortunate that at this point he finds in the task of memorizing anatomical names and spatial relationships something of a relief. The deeper questions thus evaded temporarily often go begging indefinitely. The result is a curious kind of callousness that need not be mistaken for maturity. But I suspect that the more subtle disadvantage of introducing the student to medicine by way of the cadaver is that attention is thereby attracted to *being* instead of *becoming*. Living is a state of becoming, not an unchanging finality. There are far deeper truths in the constancy of change than in the immutable permanence of death.

During the first two years of anatomy, microscopic anatomy, physiology, and the other medical sciences, the student's mind is confronted almost uninterruptedly with the uniformities of tissue structure and tissue behavior. Except for embryology, there is in most medical education throughout the world scant emphasis on life as a state of becoming: it is studied as a state of being, and its uniformities are drilled in as "laws." Until we have genetics more widely and more competently dealt with in medical schools, there will be too little attention to the almost infinite variety and uniqueness of every living thing. The means of becoming aware of the uniformities of tissue structure, form, and function is *description*—size, shape, color, and weight, measured or described.

In some countries long since, and recently in some schools in this country, the student comes in contact with patients at the very outset of his studies; that contact may tend to soften the overemphasis in the preclinical courses on rigid uniformities and similarities of form or behavior.

Following a long drill in description, the student makes, in third year, a rather abrupt discovery of the importance of narration. His clinical teachers are sure to lay an emphasis on sequences and time as related to disease processes. In the care with which it is elicited and recorded, a medical history seems to rival any instrument used for the purposes of description. I have wondered whether at about this stage medical students would not profit from having their attention called to the subject of causation—of necessary and sufficient causes; of predisposing, precipitating, and perpetuating causes; of correlation; of unique versus convergent causation. In any event, the growing importance of narration gets scant recognition as such, but is fused and confused in the growing fascination of each new subject presented by the clinicians.

Concurrently with these changes and adjustments the medical student experiences something of a conflict between the native spontaneity or initial originality he had when he first entered the medical school and the forces that bear upon him as he goes on through the four years. Though not intentionally exerted, the pressures of expectation and example tend to convert the student into a stereotype. By the end of the fourth year, medical students resemble each other in manner, thought, and behavior much more closely than in their first year. The pace of their work, the gravity of what they witness, admiration of some local figure turning

The natural history of the doctor

into imitation, the crescendo of their concern about their professional careers all increase the comfort and reassurance of losing their individual differences in conforming to a stereotype. The spontaneity, the naturalness, the self-reliance, and simplicity and homely originality of character that patients so rightly value in a doctor may or may not emerge from the eclipse. It is, I think, a close call for most medical students and young doctors: they all but prefer the protective stereotype.

But perhaps the best summary of what medical students experience is to say that they learn to take a rapidly increasing measure of responsibility. Responsibility teaches, and in medicine the penalties for not learning in time are high.

One of the experiences that greatly affect medical students in any country comes when a patient, wittingly or unwittingly, puts his life in the student's hands. I would care as little for the student who ran away from such a burden as for him who took it casually and for granted, but I'd be more afraid of the latter. But for the young man or woman on the way to professional maturity, the ultimate in responsibility is the responsibility for death due to a fault or a failure that could have been averted. There can be few honest doctors who have not at some time or other felt—or known—that they have made such a tragic error. These two experiences—human faith utterly trusting the doctor and the responsibility for a needless death—set doctors somewhat apart from other men in the special load they carry and perhaps in the special sensitiveness and clannish behavior they often show in the face of attack or criticism. Certainly there is widespread suspicion that this load of responsibility is not unrelated to the predisposition that doctors seem to show to hypertension and coronary disease, though I would myself not attribute that predisposition to any one factor.

I shall have accomplished my purpose in this chapter if I have conveyed to you how great and how strong is the demand that medical education imposes on the medical student for intellectual competence, emotional maturity, unselfishness, tenacity—and money enough to live on. Paradoxically, I shall have succeeded, too, if the impression I have given you of what the medical student goes through is both confusing and disputable. For I believe that we do not know, to the point of general agreement, much about what really happens in the life histories of medical students. Nothing would prove more valuable to the future of Great Medicine than learning steadily more of what happens in medical education. To be oriented is to know where to look for the Dawn.

Bei Fragen zur Produktsicherheit wenden Sie sich bitte an:
If you have any questions regarding product safety,
please contact:

Walter de Gruyter GmbH
Genthiner Straße 13
10785 Berlin
productsafety@degruyterbrill.com